Evaluation of the Connections to Care (C2C) Initiative

Interim Report

Lynsay Ayer, Michael Stephen Dunbar, Monique Martineau,

Clare Stevens, Dana Schultz, Wing Yi Chan, Michele Abbott,

Rebecca Weir, Harry H. Liu, Daniel Siconolfi, Vivian L. Towe

Sponsored by the Mayor's Fund to Advance New York City

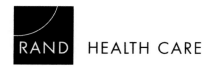

RAND HEALTH CARE

Preface

The RAND Corporation is in the process of conducting an evaluation of the Connections to Care (C2C) program, a $30 million public-private partnership that seeks to expand access to mental health services for low-income New Yorkers through community-based organizations. The C2C Collaborative—the Mayor's Fund to Advance New York City, the Mayor's Office for Economic Opportunity, and the New York City Department of Health and Mental Hygiene—partnered on this publicly and privately funded initiative. The C2C Collaborative contracted with the RAND Corporation and the McSilver Institute for Poverty Policy and Research at the New York University Silver School of Social Work for evaluation and technical assistance. This interim report presents preliminary implementation evaluation findings from data collected through March 2018, an update on impact evaluation data collection through July 2018, and a description of the approach to the cost evaluation.

This research was sponsored by the Mayor's Fund to Advance New York City under contract MFANYC_09.01.15 and carried out within the Access and Delivery Program in RAND Health Care.

RAND Health Care, a division of the RAND Corporation, promotes healthier societies by improving health care systems in the United States and other countries. We do this by providing health care decisionmakers, practitioners, and consumers with actionable, rigorous, objective evidence to support their most complex decisions.

For more information, see www.rand.org/health-care, or contact

RAND Health Care Communications
1776 Main Street
P.O. Box 2138
Santa Monica, CA 90407-2138
(310) 393-0411, ext. 7775
RAND_Health-Care@rand.org

Contents

Figures

Tables

Summary

In any given year, at least one in five adults in New York City is likely to meet the criteria for a mental health diagnosis, yet most do not receive mental health services to treat these problems (City of New York, Office of the Mayor, 2015). Problems such as depression and anxiety disproportionately affect historically underserved segments of the population, such as racial/ethnic minority and low-income individuals, that are most likely to have an unmet need for mental health services (Kataoka, Zhang, and Wells, 2002). To help close these gaps of unmet need, the Connections to Care (C2C) Collaborative—the Mayor's Fund to Advance New York City (Mayor's Fund), the Mayor's Office for Economic Opportunity, and the New York City Department of Health and Mental Hygiene—developed the C2C program. C2C is an innovative model that uses task shifting, an approach to extending evidence-informed health care skills to community-based partners, to integrate mental health support into the work of community-based organizations (CBOs) that do not focus on clinical health care. As one of New York City's ThriveNYC initiatives,[1] C2C aims to remove barriers to mental health care and, ultimately, build community resilience through responsiveness to individual and community needs.

The C2C program recognizes that mental health treatment and behavioral health interventions can involve a wide spectrum of activities to improve individual functioning and promote well-being. Such activities do not necessarily have to involve clinical treatment or occur in a clinical setting. In fact, a range of barriers, including lack of transportation, mental health stigma, and a lack of linguistic or cultural competency among clinicians, may deter some individuals from seeking care in clinical settings, where the majority of mental health services are delivered. Given additional barriers, including a shortage of trained mental health professionals and the costs of treatment that are prohibitive for many low-income populations, it is critical to build capacity in the mental health treatment system in a way that addresses these issues.

Increasing access to mental health supports in *nonclinical* settings through task shifting is an approach that may directly reduce barriers and expand access to mental health care services. In addition to decreasing logistical barriers such as transportation (clients already work with the nonclinical CBOs), this approach may also decrease the stigma people associate with seeking clinical treatment and help identify groups with mental health needs that may otherwise be missed by the mental health system. By making mental health supports available outside the clinical environment, task shifting may promote earlier needs identification and improve timely access to services that are appropriately matched to needs. In turn, this approach may reduce the

---

[1] ThriveNYC is an $850 million commitment by the City of New York to address the mental health needs of New Yorkers, launched in 2015.

adverse effects of treatable behavioral health conditions, enabling individuals to more quickly improve aspects of their quality of life, including their employment and education, and improve overall community well-being.

To build an intervention that operates through nonclinical settings, C2C integrates delivery of mental health skills into social services at 15 CBOs located throughout the city. C2C leverages the existing trusted relationships that New Yorkers already have with participating CBOs. The participating CBOs already provide a variety of services, such as career development, youth services, homeless and domestic violence services, adult education, early childhood services, and services for immigrants. Each CBO contracts with a mental health provider (MHP), developing a close, working relationship essential to ensuring the effectiveness of C2C. The MHP advises CBO staff on effective, evidence-informed interventions, while the CBO tailors the implementation of those interventions to its own context.

In C2C, CBO staff receive training, ongoing coaching, and resources to implement four initial core C2C mental health skills (hereafter, "C2C skills"): mental health screening, mental health first aid (MHFA), motivational interviewing (MI), and psychoeducation (see Table S.1 for more information). As their programs mature, CBOs may add other skills beyond these four core skills.

Core C2C Skills

Staff at CBOs participating in the C2C program receive training, coaching, and access to resources to help them deliver, at minimum, four core mental health skills.

During **mental health screening**, CBO staff screen C2C clients for conditions such as depression, anxiety, and substance use and misuse. Staff work with clients who screen positive to explain the results and identify next steps.

MHFA teaches non–mental health specialists skills to recognize and respond to signs of mental illness and substance use and misuse. C2C uses MHFA to reduce stigma, promote helping behaviors, and improve knowledge and attitudes about mental health conditions among both CBO staff and clients.

MI is a collaborative, person-centered counseling style that aims to help people make and sustain positive behavior changes. C2C uses MI to help clients change or enhance behaviors to improve their lives.

Non–mental health specialists can use **psychoeducation** to provide information to individuals with a mental health condition (and their families) to help them understand the condition and build skills to deal with it optimally. C2C uses psychoeducation to help improve mental health literacy, reduce discomfort about seeking help, and promote healthy behaviors.

As programs mature, the C2C Collaborative encourages CBOs to build on this initial set of skills by adding other appropriate context-driven skills or services to best meet the needs of staff and clients.

CBOs also develop and strengthen pathways to clinical care (e.g., through their MHP partners) that are appropriately matched to individual client needs. C2C, during its five years of operation, expects to serve up to 40,000 low-income New Yorkers (based on goals provided by participating CBOs) among its target populations: (1) young adults between the ages of 16 and 24 who are not attending school and are not employed; (2) unemployed or underemployed adults age 18 or older; and (3) parents/caregivers who are expecting or who have children four years of age or younger.

Each CBO is required to meet certain implementation requirements, such as establishing a formal relationship with an MHP, training staff members in the four core C2C mental health skills, and providing ongoing support and supervision to CBO staff to deliver core C2C skills to clients. By design, the program allots CBOs a great deal of flexibility in site-specific implementation. A CBO has the latitude to navigate its individual relationship with an MHP, set up culturally relevant training and coaching, ramp up staff readiness, and deliver the C2C supports to clients in a way that makes sense for its own organization.

The C2C program calls on both CBOs and MHPs to assume new roles that capitalize on their strengths and capabilities to increase capacity for and reduce barriers to providing mental health services. Their roles were designed so that each would learn from the other: For instance, CBOs could benefit from the mental health expertise of MHPs; in return, MHPs could learn from CBO expertise addressing social determinants of health. CBOs and MHPs become not only service providers, but also teachers who share their expertise. CBO staff leverage trusted relationships with community members and knowledge of community needs to deliver a range of mental health care supports as part of the everyday work they already do, making care more accessible. By integrating the four core C2C skills into their existing services, CBOs may gain more accurate knowledge about mental health and also expand capacity help promote mental health and well-being. C2C equips CBOs to deliver culturally responsive, evidence-informed behavioral health interventions that promote mental health and well-being and identify individuals who need more specialized care and connect them to it. MHPs support CBOs' new capabilities and skills by consulting on implementation design; performing training, ongoing coaching, and monitoring activities; applying clinical judgment to appropriately match mental health services to needs; and providing clinical care when necessary.

Working together, CBO-MHP partners identify clients' needs, select and adapt interventions, and share in both learning and quality improvement. Staff from both types of organizations may also be challenged through training and practice to confront or evolve their attitudes toward mental health issues (e.g., mental health stigma), the way mental health services are typically delivered, and who delivers them. The hope is that C2C's efforts can begin influencing community well-being more broadly, first by the diffusion of knowledge about mental health by trained CBO lay staff, who often live in the communities they serve, and second through the potential downstream effects of CBO clients who have benefited from C2C, as better supporters of their families and neighbors, or even a resource for where to get mental health support.

During the first two program years of C2C, the RAND Corporation has been working with CBOs and MHPs to provide technical assistance (with the McSilver Institute for Poverty Policy and Research at the New York University Silver School of Social Work [NYU McSilver]) and monitor the progress of the program. RAND researchers have also been collecting qualitative and quantitative data to formally evaluate the implementation, impact, and cost of C2C. This interim report describes the methods and plans for these three evaluations, provides initial findings from the implementation evaluation, and presents preliminary descriptive data from the impact evaluation. The data and analysis here derive from years 1 and 2 of C2C, though the specific time frames of data used in this report vary slightly for each evaluation, as described below.

Understanding C2C Implementation

Our implementation evaluation uses data from interviews with key leadership and staff, staff surveys, and quarterly CBO reports to describe how C2C has been implemented within and across the 15 CBOs. The implementation evaluation seeks to understand

- how the C2C program strategies were implemented (including which components were implemented and with what degree of fidelity)

- how MHPs trained and supported CBOs over time
- whether CBO staff knowledge of mental health and C2C skills, as well as attitudes and behaviors about mental health issues and services, showed improvement
- the extent to which CBOs identified clients with mental health or substance use issues as a result of C2C implementation
- the key facilitators of and barriers to effective implementation of C2C program strategies within and across CBO and MHP partnerships.

Implementation Evaluation: Key Findings

CBO-MHP Relationships
- Partnerships encountered initial cultural differences and communications challenges, but developed working relationships over time.
- Activities to build familiarity within partnerships, such as MHPs sustaining a presence on-site at CBOs, paid dividends in bridging divides.

Training
- More than 1,200 staff and supervisors were trained in at least one core C2C skill, which surpassed targets for the end of year 2.
- MHPs delivered the bulk of training, especially in year 1.
- About one year into implementation, more than two-thirds of staff were satisfied with the trainings they had received.

Coaching and Supervision
- In the 2017 staff survey, about half of staff reported receiving coaching or supervision only once or twice; a small number (6 percent) received it more than ten times.
- The C2C Collaborative updated its guidance to CBOs on these activities in May 2017 to help CBOs and MHPs develop robust ongoing coaching and supervision structures.
- Most of the 2,110 coaching hours reported between March 2016 and March 2018 were logged in year 2 of implementation.

Staff Readiness
- About half of staff surveys indicated high confidence in using a given mental health skill with a client.
- One year into implementation, trained individuals reported feeling more comfortable delivering MHFA and MI than screening or psychoeducation.
- Approximately three-quarters of staff respondents felt they had the right resources and support to deliver C2C skills and refer clients to intensive treatment when needed.

C2C Delivery
- Core C2C skills were delivered to 16,701 unique clients in the first two years, which is 98 percent of the new client target for that stage of the program.
- By the end of year 2, staff members had delivered services to an average of 70 percent of clients across CBOs.
- As of March 2018, CBOs referred 2,254 clients for mental health treatment; 60 percent of referrals resulted in at least one visit to a mental health provider (the C2C Collaborative set a goal of 70 percent of referrals resulting in at least one visit).

Early Perceptions of Impact
- Interviews indicated that staff and CBO leadership perceived a positive effect of C2C on mental health issues for clients and themselves.
- Client and staff interviewees noted changes in the way they perceive, discuss, and approach mental health issues.

The preliminary implementation findings in this interim report cover the first set of interviews and surveys—both from summer 2017—and use CBO quarterly report data from March 2016 to March 2018.

Key Implementation Evaluation Findings

CBO-MHP Relationships

One of the first implementation decisions made by all CBOs was the selection of an MHP. Some CBOs chose to partner with an organization with which they had a prior informal relationship (e.g., as a referral source). A few CBOs partnered with a provider under the same umbrella organization but with which a formal relationship did not exist; others forged a relationship with an organization with which they had never worked before. Specific implementation arrangements between CBOs and MHPs vary across organizations, including the types of CBO and MHP staff members who deliver supports, when and how supports are delivered, and the roles of each CBO and MHP with respect to training and coaching/supervision activities.

A number of sites did report some anticipated early challenges with navigating the CBO-MHP roles, including organizational culture differences and difficulties with communication between organizations. For example, MHPs were often charged with selecting and delivering training, but many initially lacked the context needed to tailor these trainings to CBO environments. In addition, while MHPs supervised CBO staff for implementation of C2C skills, they did not have the authority to require staff to attend trainings or individual coaching sessions.

CBOs and MHPs implemented several strategies to overcome these challenges, including inviting MHP staff to spend time on-site at the CBO to understand client flow and staff roles, establishing open lines of email and phone communication, scheduling structured meetings to discuss implementation and assign tasks, embedding MHP staff on-site at CBOs, specific trainings for CBO staff in the MHP intake processes, and soliciting staff feedback on training to tailor future materials. Most interviewees noted that learning about each other's organizations and keeping the lines of communication open were time-consuming but helped in building a strong relationship and a program that met the needs of clients and staff.

Training

Most training in the four core C2C skills took place either internally at the CBOs or together with MHPs, with some CBOs relying more heavily than others on MHPs to deliver training. In addition, MHFA and MI trainings were offered through external organizations, sponsored by ThriveNYC and the Mayor's Fund, respectively, and most CBOs utilized these supplemental training resources. By the end of year 2, more than 1,200 staff and supervisors had received training in at least one support, with most of that training occurring in year 1. The overall number of staff trained exceeded year 2 targets. In that same time frame, almost 250 staff and supervisors had been trained in all four core C2C skills. More than two-thirds of staff reported satisfaction with the training they received and a desire for more training. Satisfaction was associated with MHP and CBO collaboration to tailor training to a CBO's cultural context and participant population and with CBO responsiveness to staff feedback about training needs. Turnover in staff among some CBOs—a problem that preceded the start of C2C—remains a significant challenge to maintaining a sufficient number of trained staff in a handful of organizations and makes the training cycle seem continuous for some CBO leaders.

Coaching and Supervision

CBOs and MHPs developed plans for follow-up support—coaching to reinforce the four core C2C skills and supervision of trained staff—that varied according to organizational needs, site-specific implementation plans, and staff needs, availability, and capacity. Sites could engage MHP and/or CBO staff who had undergone supervisory training to provide coaching and supervision in the four core C2C skills. In the summer 2017 CBO staff survey, about half of the respondents reported receiving coaching or supervision only once or twice, and almost 20 percent reported receiving none. Conversely, a small proportion (6 percent) received coaching or supervision more than ten times. Nearly 80 percent of the 2,110 coaching hours logged by March 2018 occurred in year 2, after the C2C Collaborative issued a clarification of follow-up support requirements (coaching/supervision to be delivered on a quarterly basis, at minimum) and after CBOs and MHPs had sufficient time to develop coaching processes. MHPs delivered most of this coaching, though the proportion of CBO-administered coaching hours increased substantially by the end of year 2. Data from the next staff survey, which is currently under way, will clarify whether CBO staff continued to increase the frequency of providing coaching and supervision. As with staff perceptions of training, most CBO staff indicated both satisfaction with the supervision received and a desire for additional coaching.

Staff Readiness to Deliver C2C Skills

Among 2017 CBO staff survey respondents, about half of CBO staff trained in a given C2C skill reported high confidence in using that skill with clients. This suggests that, while many staff felt ready to use their new C2C skills in practice, a substantial proportion did not yet feel confident using them. Among individuals who had received training, respondents reported greater comfort with administering MHFA, MI, and screening than with psychoeducation; changes in C2C Collaborative-provided guidance regarding psychoeducation were issued in year 2, and most sites were in the process of responding to that guidance at the time of the survey. In interviews, some CBO staff reported feeling uncomfortable talking with their clients about mental health issues early in the implementation process, but noted that experience using C2C skills with clients and ongoing coaching and supervision helped ease that discomfort. Indeed, the majority of staff survey respondents (ranging from 70 to 85 percent) endorsed survey items regarding feeling comfortable talking about mental health issues with clients and feeling supported by their organization, as well as about having access to resources needed to help their clients and assist with referrals to more-intensive mental health treatment.

C2C Delivery

Over the first two years of the program, staff at the 15 CBOs delivered the four core C2C skills to 16,701 unique clients. The proportion of CBO clients receiving services from a CBO staff member who was trained in C2C skills rose substantially during this period, from 22 percent in year 1 to 70 percent in year 2. Many CBOs began delivering MHFA and screening in year 1, with depression as the most common mental health condition for which clients were screened. As of summer 2017, CBO direct service staff reported spending an average of more than eight hours per week delivering one or more C2C skills to clients and assisting with referrals to mental health services at the MHP or an external mental health provider. In year 2, most CBOs were implementing all four core C2C skills and began to enact more robust coaching and supervision programs to support staff in the delivery of C2C skills to clients. As of March 2018, more than 2,000 clients had been referred for mental health treatment, and almost 60 percent of those referrals were completed with at least one visit with a mental health provider. This is lower than the target set by the C2C Collaborative at the start of the project, which is to see 70 percent of referrals result in at least one visit. Although some MHPs adopted more flexible policies to accommodate C2C clients, and CBOs tried to minimize barriers to accessing more-intensive mental health treatment, some challenges remained, including client stigma; privacy concerns; and a lack of resources such as transportation, money or insurance, and child care. Future data will shed light on whether CBO-enacted strategies targeting these barriers are successful.

Perceptions of C2C Early Impact

Although we have not yet conducted a detailed assessment of client outcomes (see impact evaluation below), key informant interviews conducted thus far showed early evidence of the perception that the C2C program is having a positive effect on mental health issues (CBO [$n =$ 35] and MHP [$n = 29$] leaders, CBO staff [$n = 80$], and clients [$n = 38$]). The interviewees also indicated that C2C is creating a cultural shift in their places of work, giving them a common language with which to discuss behavioral health issues, as well as an understanding of how to approach their clients in a different way. Both CBO leaders and staff noted that trainings and C2C skill delivery also enhanced their own mental health and stress management. CBO leaders mentioned C2C's facilitation of shared resources and best practices among a wider network of like-minded organizations. Interviewees cited instances of clients benefiting from C2C skills, especially in terms of overall well-being, access to mental health resources, and stigma reduction. In addition, clients themselves shared examples of C2C's positive effects on their lives, including improved parent-child and other interpersonal relationships, improved understanding of their mental health, greater confidence, and greater access to long-term care.

Key Impact Evaluation Findings

The impact evaluation uses a client survey and other data to analyze the experiences and outcomes of participants at 13 of the 15 CBOs engaged in the C2C study and compares them with participants at ten CBOs offering similar social services but without the mental health support integration. Potential client survey participants at C2C and comparison CBO sites are screened for eligibility (i.e., fluent in English or Spanish, presence of mental health symptoms) and are enrolled if eligible and willing. Enrolled participants complete a baseline survey and follow-up surveys six and 12 months after baseline. The baseline and follow-up surveys are being completed on a rolling basis, and most participants have not yet completed follow-up surveys. The

Impact Evaluation: Key Findings

Survey Enrollment
- Eligibility screenings have been completed by 1,234 participants from C2C CBOs (805 clients) and comparison CBOs (429 clients).
- Baseline surveys have been completed by 86 percent of those eligible (634 from C2C CBOs and 267 from comparison CBOs), above the target of 80 percent of those eligible.
- Follow-up surveys will be conducted six and 12 months after baseline surveys.

Demographics (among C2C clients only)
- Most participants are over 18 years of age and from ethnic minority backgrounds.
- Over half report earning less than $5,000 per year.
- Baseline rates of moderate to severe mental health issues (depression, anxiety, alcohol/substance abuse, PTSD) ranged from 22 to 30 percent; over half report reluctance to seek mental health care.
- In the past six months, more than one-quarter had received inpatient mental health care or had seen a mental health provider.

impact evaluation aims to enroll approximately 2,000 participants in total (1,000 in each study arm) in the client survey, which is a subset of the population receiving C2C services overall.

Although the data used at this interim stage for the impact evaluation are too preliminary to draw any conclusions about the sample overall, we are able to report some descriptive characteristics of the study participants who enrolled in the evaluation between June 2017 and July 2018. Thus far, 1,234 clients have been screened from the C2C CBOs (805 clients) and the comparison CBOs (429 clients). Of those eligible, 86 percent enrolled in the study and completed baseline surveys ($n = 634$ C2C and $n = 267$ comparison participants), which exceeded the target of 80 percent of those eligible. The interim report analyses focused exclusively on the 634 clients of C2C CBOs who completed the baseline survey (i.e., not the comparison CBO participants). Most participants from the C2C CBOs were over 18 years of age and from ethnic minority backgrounds, and over half reported incomes of less than $5,000, which indicates that C2C appears to be reaching its intended target population. Baseline rates of moderate to severe mental health issues (based on previously established scoring criteria) included 22 percent for depression, 30 percent for anxiety, 20 to 30 percent for alcohol and substance abuse, and 30 percent for post-traumatic stress disorder (PTSD). Many participants expressed ambivalence about seeking mental health care in the baseline survey, and well over half endorsed statements regarding keeping feelings, emotions, or thoughts to themselves and wanting to solve problems on their own. More than one-quarter of the sample had received inpatient care for a behavioral health problem, and about the same proportion had seen a mental health provider in the past six months.

Study enrollment is expected to continue through March 2019. Until that time, more baseline surveys will be completed, and the initial study participants will begin to complete follow-up surveys. The data from these subsequent surveys will provide more information on the impact of the C2C program.

Cost Evaluation

An evaluation of the costs—and possibly overall savings—associated with C2C is also underway. The cost evaluation uses data from multiple sources to estimate the startup and maintenance costs of running the C2C program, as well as the program's effects on the cost of other social services due to improved mental health outcomes. We will collect data from financial reports submitted by CBOs to the C2C Collaborative, annual nonlabor expense and compensation reports, biannual cost surveys, assessments of participants in the impact evaluation, and administrative data from government agencies to conduct these analyses. While it is too early at this time to report on this aspect of the study, the cost evaluation will quantify the average cost of C2C per CBO on both a quarterly and yearly basis; the total cost of the C2C program (including cost of labor, payments for contracted services such as payments to MHPs, and direct and indirect costs); and the average cost per client served. RAND will also estimate the net effect of C2C on both medical spending and government expenditures at the city, state, and federal level.

Looking Ahead

At the time of this writing, CBOs and MHPs have worked together to address early implementation challenges and are focusing on full implementation of the C2C program. Over the next two years, they will continue to refine their processes and increasingly consider program sustainability. Simultaneously, we will continue our evaluations, documenting C2C implementation, impact, and cost. Implementation and cost evaluation data collection, including staff surveys, key informant interviews, and CBO program data, will continue through 2019. Impact study participant enrollment at both C2C and comparison CBO sites will continue through March 2019, with follow-up assessments ending in March 2020. A final report will be made available in 2020.

Acknowledgments

This evaluation of the C2C program was funded by the Social Innovation Fund (SIF), a program of the Corporation for National and Community Service, and by private funders. We are grateful for the efforts and partnership of the Mayor's Office for Economic Opportunity, the New York City Department of Health and Mental Hygiene, the Mayor's Fund to Advance New York City, and the McSilver Institute for Poverty Policy and Research at the New York University Silver School of Social Work. We thank Mary Acri and Joshua Breslau for their insightful comments on previous versions of this report. We also appreciate the efforts of the larger C2C evaluation team, including Susan Lovejoy, Dionne Barnes-Proby, Lisa Wagner, Emily Hoch, and Polina Kats-Kariyanakette, without whom the research could not have been conducted. The C2C program and this evaluation would not be possible without the substantial contributions of the following CBO and MHP organizations that are implementing the model (as of the end of year 2 of the program), including their staff and clients:

- Arab American Association of New York and New York University Langone Hospital–Brooklyn
- Bedford Stuyvesant Restoration Corporation and Brooklyn Community Services
- CAMBA and Jewish Board of Family and Children's Services
- Center for Employment Opportunities and CASES
- Hetrick-Martin Institute and Hetrick-Martin Institute Counseling Center
- Hudson Guild and Hudson Guild Counseling Center
- Northern Manhattan Improvement Corporation and Dean Hope Center, Teacher's College, Columbia University
- Red Hook Initiative and New York University Langone Hospital–Brooklyn
- Safe Horizon and Safe Horizon Counseling Center
- Sheltering Arms Children and Family Services and Safe Space
- STRIVE and Union Settlement and Hunter Silberman School of Social Work
- The Committee for Hispanic Children and Families and Urban Health Plan
- The Door: A Center of Alternatives and University Settlement
- The HOPE Program and Brookdale Hospital Center and Institute for Family Health
- Voces Latinas and Catholic Charities of Brooklyn and Queens.

Abbreviations

ATSPPH-SF	Attitudes Toward Seeking Professional Psychological Help Scale–Short Form
AUDIT-10	Alcohol Use Disorder Identification Test–10
BACEv2	Barriers to Access to Care Evaluation
C2C	Connections to Care
CBO	community-based organization
DAST-10	Drug Abuse Screening Test–10
DSM	Diagnostic and Statistical Manual
GAD-7	Generalized Anxiety Disorder Scale–7
GED	General Equivalency Development
K-6	Kessler 6
LES	Life Experiences Survey
MHFA	mental health first aid
MHP	mental health provider
MI	motivational interviewing
MINT	Motivational Interviewing Network of Trainers
MITI	Motivational Interviewing Treatment Integrity
NREPP	National Registry of Evidence-Based Programs and Practices
NSDUH	National Survey on Drug Use and Health
NYU McSilver	McSilver Institute for Poverty Policy and Research at the New York University Silver School of Social Work
PCL-5	PTSD Checklist for DSM–5
PHQ-8	Patient Health Questionnaire–8
PTSD	post-traumatic stress disorder
QI	quality improvement
SIF	Social Innovation Fund
THS	Trauma History Screen

WHODAS 2.0   World Health Organization Disability Assessment Schedule

WHOQOL-BREF   World Health Organization Quality of Life–BREF

1. Introduction

At least one in five adult New Yorkers is likely to meet criteria for a mental health diagnosis, yet most do not access mental health services to treat these problems (City of New York, Office of the Mayor, 2015). Mental health problems, such as depression and anxiety, disproportionately affect historically underserved segments of the population, such as racial/ethnic minority and low-income individuals. However, these groups are least likely to access mental health services (Kataoka, Zhang, and Wells, 2002). Mental health problems can range in both severity and degree of functional impairment (e.g., interference with work, school, social, and family relationships). Interventions to address these problems fall along a spectrum in terms of their goals and focus, from mental health prevention and promotion activities (i.e., enhancing mental health and preventing problems before they develop) to treatment (i.e., addressing existing mental health symptoms) (World Health Organization, 2004). If left unaddressed, mental health issues can lead to myriad negative consequences at the individual, family, and societal levels. Globally, the burden of disability related to mental health disorders overall is substantial, accounting for as much as 32 percent of the years individuals live with a disability and 13 percent of disability-adjusted life years (a measure of the effect of disability on quality of life) (Vigo, Thornicroft, and Atun, 2016). Major depression is the second-largest cause of disease burden (Vos et al., 2015). Mental health disorders are also associated with a societal cost of nearly $200 billion in lost earnings (Kessler et al., 2008). Thus, the unmet need for mental health treatment in underserved communities represents a serious public health and societal problem.

In response to this need, the Connections to Care (C2C) Collaborative—the Mayor's Fund to Advance New York City (Mayor's Fund), the Mayor's Office for Economic Opportunity (NYC Opportunity), and the New York City Department of Health and Mental Hygiene—began a publicly and privately funded initiative to expand access to mental health services among low-income, underserved communities in New York City. The Mayor's Fund, the federal Social Innovation Fund (SIF) of the Corporation for National and Community Service, the City of New York, and private donors collectively bring funding to the project.[1] C2C is one initiative of ThriveNYC, an $850 million commitment by the City of New York to address the mental health needs of New Yorkers.

---

[1] SIF was a federal grant program of the Corporation for National and Community Service that received funding from 2010 to 2016. Using public and private resources to find and grow community-based nonprofits with evidence of results, SIF intermediaries received funding to award subgrants that focus on overcoming challenges in economic opportunity, healthy futures, and youth development. The Corporation for National and Community Service awarded a SIF intermediary award to the Mayor's Fund in 2015 for use to administer the first three years of a five-year subgrant program.

In 2016, the C2C Collaborative began implementing the C2C program, an innovative model of integrating mental health support into the work of community-based organizations (CBOs) that serve low-income and at-risk populations (e.g., through workforce development, domestic violence shelters, homeless shelters, youth development, services for immigrants). Over the program's five-year span, the $30 million public-private partnership is expected to reach up to 40,000 New Yorkers through CBOs and mental health providers (MHPs). The C2C program uses a task shifting approach to maximize the capabilities of CBOs and MHPs to promote community mental health (as described in detail below). It serves clients from three target populations of low-income New Yorkers: young adults ages 16 to 24 who are not in school and are not employed, adults age 18 or older who are unemployed or underemployed, and parents/caregivers who are expecting or who have children up to the age of four. In addition to addressing immediate mental health needs, C2C and stakeholders—including the New York City government—aim to determine whether C2C strategies work as intended to remove barriers to mental health care and identify, assess, treat, and prevent mental health disorders among these populations.

Purpose of This Report

This interim report presents early qualitative and quantitative findings from the evaluation of the C2C program over the first two years of implementation. It describes the early implementation process and also presents preliminary data and information on progress for the impact evaluation. Evaluation activities will continue through March 2020. Figure 1.1 provides a high-level timeline of evaluation and data collection activities. A more detailed outline of implementation activities is included in Chapter 3.

The remainder of this introductory chapter provides background information on the problem of limited access to mental health care among low-income New Yorkers. It then describes the C2C model and the organizations involved in the implementation of the C2C program, including C2C stakeholders, CBOs, and MHPs. The chapters that follow describe the evaluation methods and initial results of the evaluation to date. The implementation chapter reports qualitative and quantitative findings thus far to describe training models and barriers and facilitators to C2C implementation. Another chapter presents preliminary descriptive data from the impact evaluation. A summary of findings and lessons learned at this interim stage of the evaluation concludes the report.

Figure 1.1. C2C Evaluation and Data Collection Timeline

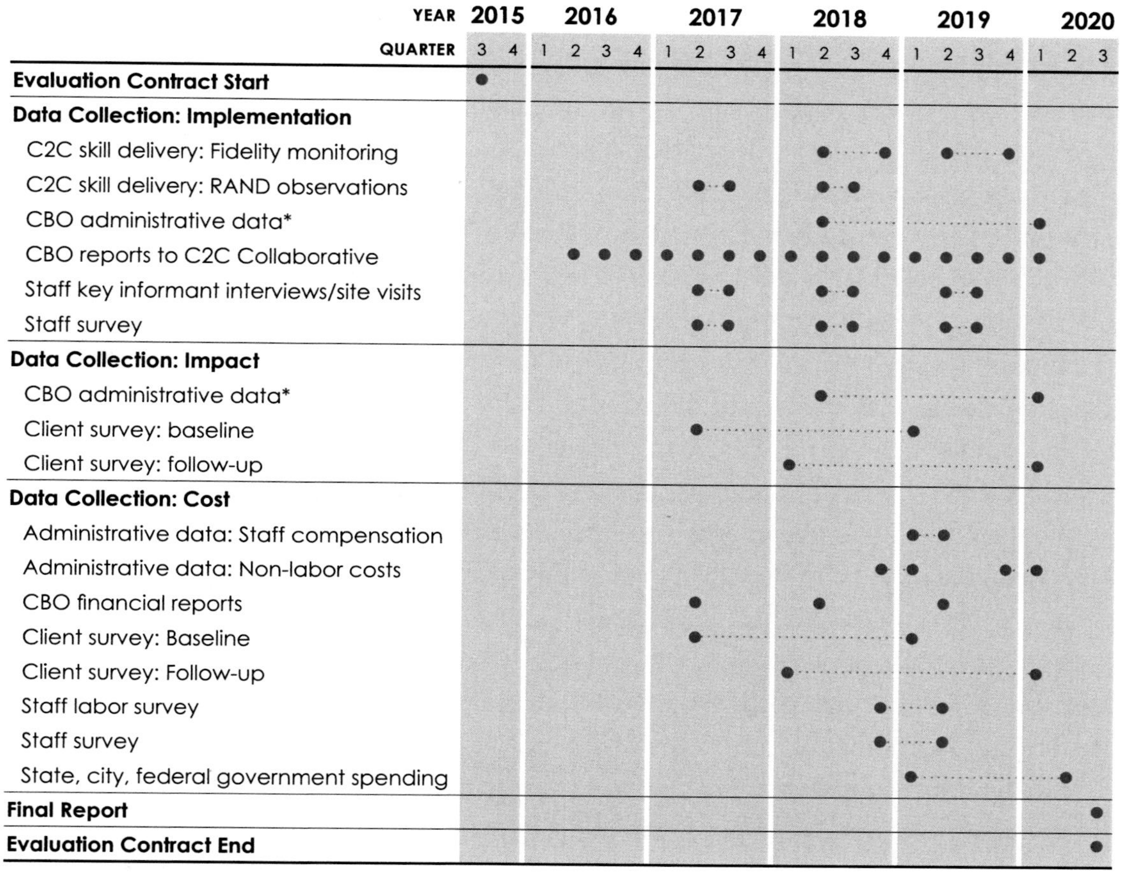

	2015		2016				2017				2018				2019				2020		
QUARTER	3	4	1	2	3	4	1	2	3	4	1	2	3	4	1	2	3	4	1	2	3
Evaluation Contract Start	●																				
Data Collection: Implementation																					
C2C skill delivery: Fidelity monitoring												●	●		●	●					
C2C skill delivery: RAND observations								●	●			●	●								
CBO administrative data*											● ┈┈┈┈┈┈┈┈┈┈┈┈┈┈┈┈┈┈┈ ●										
CBO reports to C2C Collaborative				●	●	●	●	●	●	●	●	●	●	●	●	●	●	●			
Staff key informant interviews/site visits								●	●			●	●			●	●				
Staff survey								●	●			●	●			●	●				
Data Collection: Impact																					
CBO administrative data*												● ┈┈┈┈┈┈┈┈┈┈┈┈┈┈┈┈┈ ●								
Client survey: baseline							● ┈┈┈┈┈┈┈┈┈┈┈┈┈┈┈┈┈┈┈┈┈┈ ●												
Client survey: follow-up											● ┈┈┈┈┈┈┈┈┈┈┈┈┈┈┈┈┈┈┈ ●									
Data Collection: Cost																					
Administrative data: Staff compensation																●	●				
Administrative data: Non-labor costs													●	●				●		●	
CBO financial reports							●					●				●					
Client survey: Baseline							● ┈┈┈┈┈┈┈┈┈┈┈┈┈┈┈┈┈┈┈ ●											
Client survey: Follow-up												● ┈┈┈┈┈┈┈┈┈┈┈┈┈┈┈┈┈ ●								
Staff labor survey																●	●				
Staff survey																●	●				
State, city, federal government spending																● ┈┈┈┈┈┈┈┈┈┈┈┈┈┈┈ ●					
Final Report																					●
Evaluation Contract End																					●

*Data provided by the CBO on client demographics, use of programmatic services, and mental health service use.

Background

Mental Health and Service Utilization in Low-Income Populations

Poverty is consistently linked to poor mental health and adverse outcomes (Santiago, Kaltman, and Miranda, 2013). Low-income individuals are more likely than those with higher incomes to experience chronic and acute stressors, including community violence, lack of community supports, economic and financial difficulties, and unstable housing, all of which increase the risk for mental health problems (Santiago, Kaltman, and Miranda, 2013). Despite this greater risk, most individuals living in low-income communities do not receive mental health care. A recent study analyzing nationally representative data from the National Health Interview Survey found that participants with lower incomes were 1.5 times more likely to have unmet mental health care needs than higher-income participants. In addition, those who did not have health insurance coverage were almost four times more likely to report unmet mental health needs in comparison to those with private health insurance (Roll et al., 2013).

Unmet need for mental health services is prevalent in New York City. Administrators estimate that, at any given time, over half a million adult New Yorkers have depression, yet less than 40 percent of New Yorkers report receiving mental health treatment (City of New York, Office of the Mayor, 2015), despite evidence that depression can often be treated effectively (Cuijpers, van Straten, and Warmerdam, 2007). The national rate of unmet mental health treatment needs is similar. One study found that only about 41 percent of individuals who were diagnosed with a mental health problem had received treatment in the past 12 months (Wang et al., 2005). Rates of mental health care utilization are even lower among historically underserved individuals, including racial/ethnic minority and other socioeconomically disadvantaged groups, which may contribute to or exacerbate mental health problems and other disparities, such as economic and educational inequalities (Kataoka, Zhang, and Wells, 2002).

Mental health problems such as depression, anxiety, and post-traumatic stress disorder (PTSD) often co-occur with alcohol and drug use (Mericle et al., 2012). One study found that young adults between the ages of 18 and 25 are especially vulnerable to co-occurring mental health and substance use problems (Chan, Dennis, and Funk, 2008). One reason for high rates of co-occurring disorders is that individuals with symptoms of mental health issues often turn to drugs and alcohol to help them cope with negative emotions (e.g., anger, sadness, anxiety, fear), leading to drug and alcohol addiction for some of these individuals (Metrik et al., 2016). In one study, data from two national surveys indicated rates of mental health treatment utilization of 20 percent and 11 percent, respectively, among individuals with alcohol use disorders (Edlund, Booth, and Han, 2012). Racial disparities also exist; African Americans with co-occurring mood or anxiety and substance use disorders are less likely to receive treatment for mood or anxiety disorders than their White counterparts (Hatzenbuehler et al., 2008).

Early detection of mental health problems is critical to slow or stop the progression of mental health problems and the associated costs. Recent studies have demonstrated that a positive screening for mental health problems is related to greater likelihood of mental health service utilization (Petrenko et al., 2011; Shippee et al., 2014). However, racial/ethnic minorities and individuals who are impacted by poverty are less likely to receive mental health screening in clinical settings (Hahm et al., 2015). Mental health screenings in nonclinical settings, therefore, have the potential to reduce such disparities (Thomas and Staiger, 2012). In addition, individuals who engage in substance use treatment do not always receive mental health screening, despite the fact that they are vulnerable to co-occurring mental health problems. With adequate training, substance use treatment centers can successfully implement mental health screening for youth and adults (Aitken et al., 2008; Lubman et al., 2008).

Untreated mental health problems and substance abuse can have far-reaching impacts. For example, individuals experiencing such problems may have trouble obtaining a job or achieving academic success, and they are more likely to be involved with the justice system (Watkins et al.,

2004). When symptoms become severe, those without access to mental health services often seek care from emergency rooms, a costly approach that often does not address mental health problems effectively (Ayangbayi et al., 2017). If left untreated, these problems can even be life-threatening: Depression and other mental health problems are among the strongest predictors of suicide (Gournellis et al., 2018; Krysinska and Lester, 2010), and drug and alcohol use are risk factors for accidental death and injury (Hingson and Howland, 1987; Olsson et al., 2016). Mental health conditions also confer risk for physical disability (Penninx et al., 1999) and lowered life expectancy (Chang et al., 2011). Therefore, interventions that increase engagement in mental health care, including early screening to detect problems before they become severe, could save both lives and money.

Some populations impacted by poverty may be particularly vulnerable to mental health problems. Therefore, increased access to mental health care is especially important for these groups. The three target groups of the C2C program focus on some of these populations (under- and unemployed adults, out-of-school and out-of-work youth and young adults, and expectant parents and parents/caregivers of young children).

A recent study analyzing population-based survey data from Australia, the United States, the United Kingdom, and Germany found that a few months of unemployment can have negative consequences on mental health (Cygan-Rehm, Kuehnle, and Oberfichtner, 2017). Unemployed adults face barriers to care as they struggle with mental health problems. Among those who are underemployed, mental health services are also often out of reach. The typical structure of mental health services (e.g., weekly visits, weekday appointments) makes it difficult for those who work on a shift schedule and those who do not own a car to use mental health care (Anderson et al., 2017; Santiago, Kaltman, and Miranda, 2013).

Another vulnerable group of low-income individuals that the C2C program seeks to help is out-of-school and out-of-work youth. Youth who have dropped out of high school are more likely to be depressed and to have attempted suicide than high school graduates (Liem, Lustig, and Dillon, 2010; Maynard, Salas-Wright, and Vaughn, 2015). In addition, out-of-school adolescents and young adults are more affected by lack of access to health insurance than their student counterparts (Cadigan, Lee, and Larimer, 2018).

Expectant mothers and caregivers are particularly vulnerable to depression during pregnancy and the postpartum period because of hormonal changes and stressors associated with childbirth and child rearing (Brummelte and Galea, 2010; Cunningham and Zayas, 2002). Expectant parents and caregivers with young children who have low incomes report higher rates of mental health problems—and are less likely to seek mental health treatment—than those with higher incomes (Lazear et al., 2008). Many note that a fear of losing custody of their children is a barrier to seeking care (Anderson et al., 2006). In addition, competing priorities such as childcare and their children's mental health needs can add to the challenge of participating in their own mental health services (Anderson et al., 2006). The bidirectional relationship between maternal and child mental health makes providing mental health services to parents especially important, as better parental well-being is related to more positive mental and behavioral health in children (Kvalevaag et al., 2013; Zalewski et al., 2017).

Mental Health Treatment Capacity

Evidence-based interventions, such as cognitive behavioral therapy, are generally effective in treating a wide range of mental health problems, including depression, anxiety, and PTSD (Bisson et al., 2007; Hofmann and Smits, 2008; Miranda et al., 2003; Roy-Byrne et al., 2010; Shear et al., 2005). Unfortunately, there is a critical shortage of mental health providers who can deliver such interventions. One in five counties in the United States has an unmet need for mental health professionals (Thomas et al., 2009). The need for psychiatrists is even greater: 96 percent of the nation's 3,140 counties do not have adequate access to psychiatric services (Thomas et al., 2009). In addition, not all clinicians have access to the training and supervision needed to deliver evidence-based treatments. Consequently, regions across all income strata are trying to strategize on how to fill such workforce gaps, including the exploration of new delivery models, many of which leverage nonspecialist health workers (American Hospital Association, 2016; Kazdin and Rabbitt, 2013).

Barriers to Mental Health Care for Low-Income Adults and Youth

Research has revealed that there are many barriers to accessing mental health services. These barriers can be categorized into two groups: non–stigma-related (i.e., logistical) and stigma-related (Clement et al., 2012). Non–stigma-related barriers—also seen as "logistical" barriers—to mental health care include cost, lack of health insurance or inadequate insurance, limited availability of mental health providers (e.g., due to a shortage of providers in a given region), lack of transportation, inflexible mental health services, previous negative experience with mental health care, lack of culturally and/or linguistically appropriate care, and mistrust of the health care system (Santiago, Kaltman, and Miranda, 2013). Some of these barriers (e.g., cost, lack of health insurance and transportation) disproportionately affect low-income communities. Mental health stigma refers to "the stigma and discrimination that individuals believe to be associated with receiving care for a mental health problem" (Clement et al., 2012). Stigma-related barriers include individuals' concerns about the potential negative consequences associated with seeking treatment for a mental health problem. For example, someone in need of mental health care may avoid seeking it due to shame, embarrassment, or fear that others would find out about seeking treatment (Hadfield and Wittkowski, 2017; Lazear et al., 2008). C2C is designed to address both stigma- and non–stigma-related barriers.

Mental Health Task Shifting

To broaden access to mental health support and address many of the aforementioned logistical and stigma-related barriers to mental health care, C2C implements a model of service delivery known as "task shifting" or "task sharing."[2] In the context of mental health, task shifting is a way of expanding the mental health workforce by training lay staff to deliver basic mental health screening and evidence-informed psychosocial intervention strategies (Chibanda et al., 2011; Govindarajan and Ramamurti, 2018; Huang et al., 2014; Legha et al., 2015). Under this model, mental health specialists (e.g., psychiatrists, psychologists, social workers) provide training, supervision, and fidelity monitoring for nonspecialists (e.g., community outreach and early childhood workers, teachers, employment specialists, shelter staff) over the course of the intervention. Training nonspecialists to deliver mental health interventions through trusted CBOs has the potential to increase mental health access among underserved populations by expanding the mental health workforce and integrating mental health supports and interventions that are culturally competent, are accessible, and lack the stigma associated with formal mental health clinics. Evidence has shown that task shifting enables referrals, detection of mental health issues, psychoeducation, and follow-up care with positive outcomes for clients (Kakuma et al., 2011).

Integrating mental health support into community-based settings also has the potential to improve the usual services delivered by CBOs, as well as the overall health care system (Patel et al., 2013). For example, a CBO that focuses on job training and workforce development may find that clients' mental health and substance use issues are barriers to program participation and successful employment outcomes. When they are able to identify and address clients' mental health concerns swiftly, CBOs may find that their clients are better able to participate in programs and ultimately better prepared for employment. With mental health supports delivered by nonspecialists, task shifting could also improve the efficiency of the mental health care system, allowing mental health professionals to focus their time on delivering specialty care to those who need it.

The concept of task shifting emerged from global health initiatives that focused on disease prevention and treatment. Task shifting has been adopted in mental health because of its ability to be scaled up to provide services to individuals with limited access to care as well as its adaptability to diverse cultures and local conditions (dos Santos et al., 2016; Kazdin and Rabbitt, 2013; Matsuzaka et al., 2017). Several factors have been hypothesized to increase the likelihood of success of mental health task shifting interventions: (1) assessment and integration of local context into the intervention; (2) referral and care pathways that follow a protocol to address a mental health issue and achieve a specific health goal; (3) access to training, ongoing supervision, and decision supports that help lay workers know when to take action and which actions to take; (4) integration of quality improvement (QI) practices that allow for assessment and rapid improvement of care; and (5) planning for capacity building and sustainability (Belkin et al., 2011). The C2C initiative incorporates these elements and seeks to build on the current

---

[2] Some researchers, practitioners, and policymakers use the term "task sharing" to reflect that tasks may remain shared between the specialist and lay providers. In this report, we use "task shifting," as it is the more commonly used term, but many of the C2C models implemented by CBOs and MHPs may be best described as "task sharing."

evidence that lay staff can effectively deliver mental health interventions, as well as inform further use and implementation of the model in New York City.

While the specific combined package of the four C2C skills has not yet been studied, the individual skills (screening for detection of mental health conditions, motivational interviewing [MI], mental health first aid [MHFA], and psychoeducation) have independently been shown to be effective on a range of outcomes (e.g., substance use and misuse, depression symptoms) when delivered by trained lay people (Acri et al., 2015; Acri et al., 2014; Barrowclough et al., 2001; Cunningham et al., 2012; de Roten et al., 2013; Hohmna, Doran, and Koutsenok, 2009; Jensen et al., 2011; Kagee et al., 2013; Schwalbe, Oh, and Zweben, 2014; Smith et al., 2012; Wong, Collins, and Cerully, 2015). International research in resource-limited settings also indicates that other mental health interventions delivered by nonspecialist lay workers can produce positive outcomes, such as decreased depression, reduced PTSD symptoms, decreased alcohol consumption, and reduced stigma (Bolton et al., 2003; van Ginneken et al., 2013). Further, studies suggest that because known lay staff are viewed as more credible and trustworthy than unfamiliar mental health professionals, engagement in mental health treatment is improved when known lay staff perform some tasks of care (Gopalan et al., 2010).

Other programs have applied mental health task shifting to primary care medical settings (Patel et al., 2013). For example, lay staff provided depression screening and psychoeducation in primary care sites in two underserved communities in Los Angeles (Chung et al., 2010). A randomized controlled trial found that men who received the collaborative depression care, including from nonclinical staff, reported better mental wellness and fewer hospital visits than those who received usual care (Mehta et al., 2017).

The evaluation of C2C will help describe the different ways the program is implemented by CBOs and will help determine whether and how mental health task shifting through CBOs and MHPs can address low-income individuals' mental health and other outcomes (RAND Corporation, 2017). As trusted entities familiar to their surrounding communities and client populations, CBOs may be an ideal setting for delivering mental health supports. C2C also recognizes that some clients will need access to stepped, specialty mental health care; to facilitate this, C2C enables and funds CBOs to partner with MHPs. Together, CBOs and MHPs develop and strengthen referral pathways to promote access to stepped care for clients in need of a higher level of care. CBOs can partner with culturally responsive MHPs; where that is not possible, CBOs may be able to leverage their expertise in culturally responsive services to build the cultural skills of MHP staff. Meanwhile, MHPs provide ongoing support and guidance for CBO staff through supervision and coaching.

Connections to Care

C2C brings together many stakeholders and partners toward the goal of increasing awareness of mental health needs, access to services, and community-based provision of services. In fall

2015 and winter 2016, the C2C Collaborative used a competitive process to choose 15 CBOs operating throughout New York City to participate in the C2C program. The 15 CBOs each applied with an MHP organization licensed to deliver professional mental health services in New York City. The type of CBO-MHP relationship varies by organization, and the term "relationship" or "partnership" is used colloquially to refer to those arrangements. In most cases, a third-party MHP was contracted by the CBO to provide training, technical assistance (often in the form of "coaching and supervision" of mental health support skills), and direct services to the CBO. In other cases, the CBO had an existing mental health clinic within its agency that was engaged as the MHP to provide services where they otherwise were not occurring within the CBO social service settings.

The chosen CBOs provide a wide range of services to their clients, including workforce development, youth-oriented programming, immigration services, HIV testing, early childhood education, homeless shelters, and domestic violence interventions. As summarized previously, C2C programming is focused on CBO clients from three target populations of low-income New Yorkers: young adults ages 16 to 24 who are not in school and are not employed; adults age 18 or older who are not employed or are underemployed; and caregivers and parents who are expecting or who have children up to the age of four.

Our evaluation of C2C examines the program through three separate but related lenses:

1. **Implementation:** This focuses on the C2C skills and referral processes implemented within and across CBOs; how C2C implementation affected CBO clients' access to a range of mental health promotion, treatment, and illness prevention services (including clients who do and do not screen positive for a mental health condition); the facilitators of and barriers to C2C implementation, including characteristics of both CBOs and MHPs; and whether CBO staff trained in one or more of the C2C skills exhibited improved knowledge, behaviors, and attitudes about mental health issues and services.
2. **Program impact:** This examines the extent to which C2C improved participants' access to mental health care and well-being on a variety of outcomes.
3. **Program cost:** This focuses on the resources required to set up and maintain the C2C program, the program's impact on participants' health care spending and government outlays (i.e., whether the program can generate savings for the city and state governments of New York and the federal government), and the program's potential cost impact on CBOs and MHPs.

Intervention Model

The C2C Collaborative has partnered with national and local funders to support the selected CBOs and their MHPs to incorporate four evidence-informed mental health skills into daily CBO programming to improve outcomes at the program and individual levels. The ultimate goals of the C2C program are to promote the well-being and mental health of program participants by increasing client access to and improving CBO capacity for delivery of evidence-informed mental health supports. The evaluation also seeks to understand how C2C can promote mental health, prevent mental health problems from developing or worsening, and improve mental health outcomes overall. For long-term changes to occur, several early and intermediate steps must happen first. The early phase of C2C focuses on providing staff at CBOs with the four core mental health skills (screening for common mental health and substance use and misuse disorders, MI, MHFA, and psychoeducation). Using this task shifting approach, staff use these skills to identify their clients' unmet mental health needs. As CBO staff use their new skills (with supervision and coaching provided by the MHP), they will be able to address many of their clients' mental health needs and provide a warm hand-off to mental health providers for more serious issues. The MHP remains connected with the CBO after the initial trainings and throughout implementation to continue promoting task shifting through ongoing coaching, monitoring, and support.

C2C is not intended to be a substitute for professional mental health services (e.g., psychological evaluation for diagnostic purposes; psychotherapy delivered by clinical psychologist, licensed clinical social worker, counselor, psychiatrist). Instead, the program is designed to make it more likely that people in need of clinical care will get it by preparing them for engagement and retention in such services (e.g., by reducing stigma and other barriers to care). Ultimately, the C2C program is designed to address a wide range of unmet mental health needs, thus improving outcomes for individuals served. CBO staff can also apply the person-centered conversation skills and strategies they develop through C2C to improve the everyday, non–mental health–related conversations they have with the participants they serve.

Figure 1.2 presents a logic model that connects inputs (C2C actors, such as funders, the C2C Collaborative, CBOs and their MHPs, and resources); C2C program strategies (mental health supports and referrals); outputs ("products" delivered by implementing C2C program strategies); and intended outcomes at the individual, program, and systems levels. The content of this logic model is consistent with both C2C-specific goals and current literature on best practices in implementing sustainable, evidence-based practices in community settings (Aarons, Hurlburt, and Horwitz, 2011; Scheirer and Dearing, 2011). The logic model was developed through an iterative process involving RAND and the C2C Collaborative.

Inputs are all participants, community assets, and resources, including programs and policies that can support program implementation or client access to mental health services. Consistent with current best practices on creating sustainable impacts on complex health challenges, C2C brings together a breadth of partners from multiple sectors, including those outside the health system (Erickson and Andrews, 2011). Collaboration from such a group of partners can lead to more community-driven ways of solving health challenges, the buy-in needed to sustain such changes, and the political will to enact policy changes that ultimately lead to wider and longer-lasting change (Towe et al., 2016). This multisectoral group of C2C partners will support a set of strategies to reach the desired C2C outcomes.

The C2C program strategies include a range of activities to promote the integration of new mental health skills and services into routine CBO work, including the four core C2C skills, as well as referral pathways between the CBO and MHP. C2C's core set of mental health skills was

10

Figure 1.2. C2C Program Logic Model

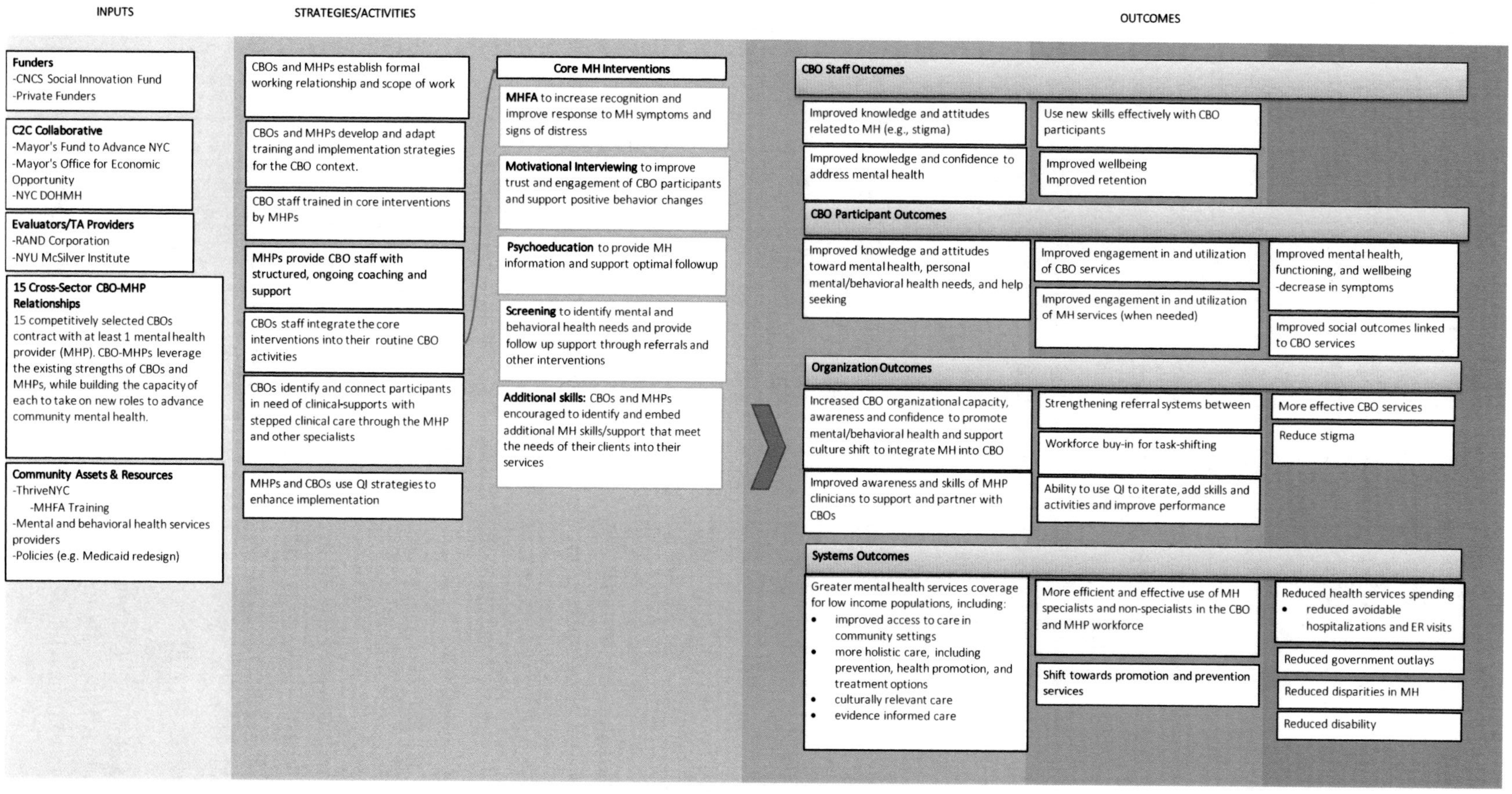

INPUTS

Funders
-CNCS Social Innovation Fund
-Private Funders

C2C Collaborative
-Mayor's Fund to Advance NYC
-Mayor's Office for Economic Opportunity
-NYC DOHMH

Evaluators/TA Providers
-RAND Corporation
-NYU McSilver Institute

15 Cross-Sector CBO-MHP Relationships
15 competitively selected CBOs contract with at least 1 mental health provider (MHP). CBO-MHPs leverage the existing strengths of CBOs and MHPs, while building the capacity of each to take on new roles to advance community mental health.

Community Assets & Resources
-ThriveNYC
-MHFA Training
-Mental and behavioral health services providers
-Policies (e.g. Medicaid redesign)

STRATEGIES/ACTIVITIES

CBOs and MHPs establish formal working relationship and scope of work

CBOs and MHPs develop and adapt training and implementation strategies for the CBO context.

CBO staff trained in core interventions by MHPs

MHPs provide CBO staff with structured, ongoing coaching and support

CBOs staff integrate the core interventions into their routine CBO activities

CBOs identify and connect participants in need of clinical supports with stepped clinical care through the MHP and other specialists

MHPs and CBOs use QI strategies to enhance implementation

Core MH Interventions

MHFA to increase recognition and improve response to MH symptoms and signs of distress

Motivational Interviewing to improve trust and engagement of CBO participants and support positive behavior changes

Psychoeducation to provide MH information and support optimal followup

Screening to identify mental and behavioral health needs and provide follow up support through referrals and other interventions

Additional skills: CBOs and MHPs encouraged to identify and embed additional MH skills/support that meet the needs of their clients into their services

OUTCOMES

CBO Staff Outcomes

Improved knowledge and attitudes related to MH (e.g., stigma)

Improved knowledge and confidence to address mental health

Use new skills effectively with CBO participants

Improved wellbeing
Improved retention

CBO Participant Outcomes

Improved knowledge and attitudes toward mental health, personal mental/behavioral health needs, and help seeking

Improved engagement in and utilization of CBO services

Improved engagement in and utilization of MH services (when needed)

Improved mental health, functioning, and wellbeing
-decrease in symptoms

Improved social outcomes linked to CBO services

Organization Outcomes

Increased CBO organizational capacity, awareness and confidence to promote mental/behavioral health and support culture shift to integrate MH into CBO

Improved awareness and skills of MHP clinicians to support and partner with CBOs

Strengthening referral systems between CBO and MHP

Workforce buy-in for task-shifting

Ability to use QI to iterate, add skills and activities and improve performance

More effective CBO services

Reduce stigma

Systems Outcomes

Greater mental health services coverage for low income populations, including:
- improved access to care in community settings
- more holistic care, including prevention, health promotion, and treatment options
- culturally relevant care
- evidence informed care

More efficient and effective use of MH specialists and non-specialists in the CBO and MHP workforce

Shift towards promotion and prevention services

Reduced health services spending
  reduced avoidable hospitalizations and ER visits

Reduced government outlays

Reduced disparities in MH

Reduced disability

NOTE: CNCS = Corporation for National and Community Service; DOHMH = Department of Health and Mental Hygiene.

11

selected from an array of possible approaches based on evidence of each of the supports to affect positive change on mental health outcomes and to be implemented by individuals without specialized (e.g., clinical) training in mental health care delivery. As the program matures, the C2C Collaborative encourages participating organizations to build upon this initial set of skills through the addition of other context-driven skills or services that can be implemented by non–mental health specialists with the right supports.

Another key C2C strategy is the implementation of a systematic and ongoing QI process to assess and continually enhance outcomes for program participants. While participating organizations entered the program with varying levels of experience implementing QI strategies, the C2C Collaborative has provided technical assistance on key components, including setting program goals and targets; systematically collecting and reviewing data to gauge progress; interpretation of program data; and using data to make targeted, informed choices about program changes or enhancements. The use of QI techniques will continue to be a focus of technical assistance and program implementation in the next three years of C2C.

C2C Outcomes

C2C implementation is expected to produce staff-, participant-, organization-, and system-level outcomes. Many, but not all, outcomes, are investigated in the C2C evaluation. Specific evaluation research questions and outcome measures are described in the next chapter.

At the CBO staff level, C2C is expected to

- improve knowledge and attitudes related to mental health (e.g., stigma)
- improve knowledge and confidence to address mental health
- increase use of new C2C skills with CBO participants
- improve staff well-being and retention
- facilitate the use of QI methods to focus and improve the impact of the incorporated skills and methods, and to further expand upon them.

At the participant level, C2C aims to demonstrate that implementation of C2C program strategies into CBO workflows can

- improve participants' knowledge and attitudes about mental health issues
- improve engagement in and use of CBO services
- increase engagement in and use of mental health services, when needed
- improve mental health outcomes and general functioning of participants
- increase participants' ability to achieve other targeted program-specific outcomes in areas such as education, housing stability, and employment.

At the organizational level, C2C is expected to

- increase capacity, awareness, and confidence to promote mental health care and support an organizational culture shift to integrate mental health awareness
- improve awareness and skills of MHP clinicians to support and partner with CBOs
- strengthen referral systems between CBOs and MHPs

- improve buy-in (at both CBOs and MHPs) for task shifting
- improve ability to use QI techniques
- provide more effective general CBO services
- reduce stigma.

System-level outcomes of C2C are expected to include

- greater mental health services coverage for low-income populations
- more efficient and effective use of mental health specialists and nonspecialists in MHPs and CBOs
- shift in focus toward promotion and prevention services
- increased presence of MHPs in communities and an increase in MHPs partnering with CBOs to meet needs
- increased capacity of the mental health workforce to provide culturally competent care
- reduced health services spending and government outlays
- reduced mental health disparities
- reduced disability.

As described above, CBO staff receive training, ongoing coaching, and support from their MHP to implement, at minimum, four core C2C mental health skills: mental health screening, MHFA, MI, and psychoeducation.

- **Mental health screenings** for common mental health and substance use and misuse issues are often used to determine the level and type of additional supports or services that a client needs. In low-income settings, there is emerging evidence that screenings for mental health issues—conducted by nonclinical staff who have undergone adequate training—result in population-level gains, including greater mental health services coverage, more effective use of health care staff and resources, and reductions in stigma (Kagee et al., 2013). This appears to be especially true when there is also a clear referral strategy in place for individuals who screen positive for common mental health issues (Kagee et al., 2013), as offered through C2C. The C2C model specified that CBOs must screen clients for depression, anxiety, and substance use and misuse; additional screenings could be added at the discretion of the CBO.
- **MHFA** was designed specifically for use by lay people and non–mental health specialists. The behavioral health problems covered in MHFA trainings include depression; anxiety; other psychiatric disorders (e.g., schizophrenia, eating disorders); and substance use disorders. The objective of MHFA training is to facilitate trainees' ability to identify and respond to clients' behavioral health problems. More specifically, MHFA training is intended to (1) increase awareness of signs and symptoms of behavioral health problems, including mental health problems and substance use; (2) enhance active listening skills; and (3) provide skills in immediate intervention, crisis response, and referrals to mental health services. To support these skills, MHFA training also seeks to build trainees' mental health literacy (knowledge and vocabulary) and normalize and destigmatize mental health problems. MHFA has been found to be effective for improving trainees' knowledge and attitudes and for promoting helping behavior toward individuals with mental health disorders and/or symptoms (Wong, Collins, and Cerully, 2015). Several studies support the effectiveness of MHFA in

improving recognition of mental health symptoms, knowledge of mental health support and treatment resources, attitudes about social distance, and confidence in providing help by staff trained in MHFA (Wong, Collins, and Cerully, 2015).

- **MI** is a collaborative, person-centered method of helping clients to explore and resolve ambivalence about their behavior, and to elicit and enhance motivation to change behavior (Miller and Rollnick, 2008). Originally developed in the context of substance use treatment, multiple studies have demonstrated the effectiveness of MI in changing behaviors related to a variety of health and mental health issues (Lundahl and Burke, 2009). MI has been used effectively to facilitate behavior change in multiple medical and psychiatric conditions, including anxiety, depression, and PTSD (Burke, Arkowitz, and Menchola, 2003); comorbid psychiatric and substance use and misuse issues; and a wide range of other issues that affect well-being. For example, MI has been applied in education settings to improve a range of behaviors that include (but are not limited to) dropout rates, marijuana use, and obesity. MI has also been increasingly applied in corrections settings (Miller and Rollnick, 2013). There is moderate evidence to suggest that non–mental health professionals can be trained in MI and implement it with fidelity. Mental health and non–mental health professionals alike are most likely to develop MI skillfulness through opportunities for continued learning over time, especially coaching that includes individualized feedback based on observed practice (Miller and Rollnick, 2013; Schwalb, Oh, and Zweben, 2014).
- **Psychoeducation** integrates education and strengths-based therapeutic interventions to empower people to improve their mental health and well-being. Psychoeducation includes providing accurate information about mental health issues and helping participants develop new tools and competencies to manage mental health conditions and other challenges in optimal ways. It can be delivered in group or individual settings, and it may target individuals affected by or at risk for mental health issues or their families. Psychoeducation is a flexible mental health support that has shown potential utility when incorporated into treatment programs for a range of mental health and related problems (e.g., severe mental illness, adjustment to medical diagnoses; Lukens and McFarlane, 2004; Pekkala and Merinder, 2002). In addition, there is emerging evidence that lay providers can successfully deliver psychoeducation. Individuals in India diagnosed with schizophrenia who received psychoeducation from lay health workers combined with usual care showed increased adherence to medications after 12 months in comparison to participants in the usual care group (Chatterjee et al., 2014).

While the C2C model requires that some combination of staff at each CBO receive training in all four skills, each CBO has developed a customized plan for incorporating these modalities into their existing services. Not every staff member must be trained in and deliver all four C2C skills, and skills can be delivered by a combination of staff members as appropriate. Not all clients will receive all four supports, and clients can receive a different mix of C2C skills in an order that best serves client needs and each CBO's implementation plan.

In addition to the adoption of the C2C skills described above, each CBO and its MHP are expected to develop and strengthen referral pathways from the CBO to the MHP with clients who request or agree to additional care. The CBO is expected to work with the MHP to ensure that clients receive services and to follow up with clients about appointments and their progress.

Streamlining the referral process and maximizing hand-offs to MHP providers who have training and licensure to provide specialized clinical care is particularly important for low-income individuals in need of treatment, as they face numerous barriers to accessing quality care.

2. Evaluation Methods

In this section, we briefly describe the goals and methods of evaluation of the C2C program in three parts: the implementation, the impact, and the cost of C2C. Table 2.1 provides an overview of the key individual- and program-level domains to be measured for each evaluation component. The measures described in this chapter are limited to those most relevant to this interim report (see Appendix A for more detail about the measures for each evaluation).

Table 2.1. Outcome Measurement Domains by Evaluation and Type

	Individual-Level Outcome Measurement Domains	Program-Level Outcome Measurement Domains
Implementation Evaluation		**Annual key informant interviews/site visits** • Implementation fidelity: perceived use of C2C modalities with clients • Partnership collaboration: partnership interaction, clarity on roles and responsibilities, collaborative decisionmaking • Participant engagement in C2C program strategies: psychosocial barriers, logistical barriers, effective solutions • Implementation facilitators and barriers: CBO and MHP leadership and staff perspectives • Participant attitudes toward the C2C program and satisfaction with C2C services • CBO staff job satisfaction, and attitudes toward and satisfaction with the C2C program **Annual supervisor ratings of CBO staff delivering C2C modalities** • Treatment (screening, MI, MHFA, and psychoeducation) fidelity: CBO staff delivering C2C modalities with fidelity **Annual RAND observations of CBO staff delivering C2C modalities** • Treatment (screening, MI, MHFA, and psychoeducation) fidelity: CBO staff delivering C2C modalities with fidelity **Quarterly reports** • Treatment (screening, MI, MHFA, and psychoeducation) fidelity: training of CBO staff in C2C modalities • Implementation fidelity: adherence to C2C program procedures • Service delivery: number of CBO clients receiving each C2C modality, percentage of target receiving each modality • Continuous QI: customized indicators for each CBO **Annual staff surveys**

Individual-Level Outcome Measurement Domains	Program-Level Outcome Measurement Domains
	• Implementation fidelity: perceived use of C2C modalities with clients • Treatment (screening, MI, MHFA, and psychoeducation) fidelity: training of CBO staff • Knowledge (e.g., mental health/substance use an misuse symptoms, problems, treatment, C2C modalities) • Attitudes (e.g., perceptions of mental health problems, evidence-based practice, stigma, social distance, beliefs about treatment) • Behavior (e.g., readiness to help, confidence, intentions to help, help provided) • Organizational climate (e.g., mission, communication, and change), perceived organizational support, and job stress. **CBO data management systems** • Treatment (screening, MI, MHFA, and psychoeducation) fidelity: delivery of evidence-based mental health modality as designed • Implementation fidelity: adherence to C2C program procedures • Client engagement in C2C program strategies: CBO program types associated with client engagement in C2C program strategies

Impact Evaluation	**Participant baseline and follow-up assessments** • Functioning (e.g., quality of life, disability) • Stressful experiences • Mental health symptoms (e.g., depression, anxiety, PTSD) • Drug/alcohol misuse/dependence • Barriers to accessing mental health care • Readiness to engage in mental health care • Mental health service utilization (including C2C services) **Administrative data** • Health services (e.g., psychiatric hospitalizations and emergencies) • Housing • Mental health service use (e.g., referral to mental health care, treatment uptake, dosage) • Employment (e.g., employment rate, job retention, receipt of unemployment benefits) • Education (e.g., absenteeism, post-secondary education)	

	Individual-Level Outcome Measurement Domains	Program-Level Outcome Measurement Domains
Cost Evaluation	**Participant baseline and follow-up assessments** • Program participation (e.g., time spent on program) • Out-of-pocket payments for medical services • Employment status and employment income • Time spent in substance abuse treatment facilities (e.g., number of months) • Time spent in jail (e.g., number of months) • Government benefits received (e.g., unemployment benefits, housing subsidies, food stamps) **Administrative data** • Medical expenditures (e.g., medical claims from the Medicaid agency) • Government expenditures (e.g., expenses on food stamps, housing subsidies, unemployment benefits)	**CBO/MHP labor input** • Number of days spent on C2C-related activities **Administrative data** • Labor cost (e.g., annual staff salaries and fringe benefits) • Nonlabor cost (e.g., computer hardware and software; rent, utilities, supplies, and transportation; overhead) • Direct C2C-related payments to vendors (including MHPs)

Implementation Evaluation

The goals of the C2C implementation evaluation are to examine how C2C is implemented within and across CBOs; whether CBO staff exhibit improved knowledge, behaviors, and attitudes about mental health issues and services; how C2C implementation changes CBO client access to mental health services; and the facilitators of and barriers to C2C implementation. The main research questions are

1. How were the C2C program strategies implemented, including which components were implemented and with what degree of fidelity?
2. How did the MHPs train and support the CBOs to implement C2C program strategies over time?
3. Do CBO staff have improved knowledge of mental health and C2C modalities, as well as attitudes and behaviors about mental health issues and services?
4. To what extent have the CBOs identified clients with mental health or substance use and misuse issues as a result of C2C implementation?
5. What are the key facilitators of and barriers to effective implementation of C2C program strategies within and across CBO and MHP partnerships?

The implementation evaluation uses a mixed-method approach (i.e., collecting qualitative and quantitative data) and prospective design (i.e., follows the same group over time and includes multiple assessment waves over time). The primary data sources for the implementation evaluation findings described in this report are (1) annual key informant interviews with CBO and MHP leadership and staff, as well as with CBO clients who have participated in C2C; (2)

annual staff surveys; and (3) CBO quarterly reports. A detailed description of the measures used is included in Appendix A.

Key Informant Interviews

We conducted key informant interviews during summer 2017 as a part of annual site visits to all 15 CBOs to collect qualitative data on program implementation from a variety of stakeholders. During each of these 15 site visits, we interviewed CBO leaders (e.g., CBO executive directors, CBO C2C program directors), MHP leaders (e.g., MHP clinical directors, MHP counselors), and CBO frontline staff (e.g., staff trained in and providing C2C skills to CBO clients). We interviewed a total of 35 CBO leaders, 29 MHP leaders, and 80 participating CBO frontline staff. Leadership and frontline staff interviewees included organizational leaders and program managers, psychologists, social workers, client intake specialists, case managers, job counselors, and life skills instructors, among others. At 12 of 15 sites, we interviewed at least one CBO client who had been offered and/or received C2C skills, reaching a total of 38 CBO clients. The interview protocols for program staff covered a range of topics, including overall program implementation, intervention fidelity, attitudes toward C2C, job satisfaction, collaboration with partners, and implementation barriers and facilitators. The interview protocols for program participants covered experiences with and attitudes toward the program.

Annual Staff Survey

We conducted the first wave of annual staff surveys in the summer of 2017 (early year 2) to gain a broader perspective on program implementation from the perspective of different types of program staff. CBO staff who had ever received training in any of the four core C2C skills and who were still actively working at the CBO with a valid email address were eligible to participate. A total of 140 CBO staff members responded to the survey (response rate of 34 percent). Approximately half (52 percent) of respondents were direct service providers (e.g., counselors, educators, service coordinators); 27 percent were leadership, management or supervisors; and 21 percent were administrative or other staff (e.g., security, receptionist). Most of the sample (62 percent) had been involved with the organization for between one and five years; 15 percent had been with the organization for less than one year, and 23 percent had been involved for more than five years. Staff surveys were brief and covered topics such as staff experiences with C2C training and service delivery, confidence in one's ability to administer C2C skills, knowledge about mental health issues, organizational climate and perceived organization supportiveness, and staff use of specific resources and strategies during client interactions.

CBO Quarterly Reports

All 15 CBOs provide aggregate quarterly data to the Mayor's Fund. Data used for this interim report came from years 1 and 2 of program implementation. These data included participant demographics and key program services and outcomes, including program performance against targets and other aspects of program and contract management.

In this interim report, we examine findings from the first wave of key informant interviews and staff surveys (from in summer 2017) as well as CBO quarterly report data from the first two years of C2C implementation (March 2016–March 2018). At the time of this writing, the second wave of key informant interviews and staff surveys are under way; the final report will describe findings from those efforts, including changes in implementation from wave 1 to wave 2.

Impact Evaluation

The goal of the C2C impact evaluation is to examine the effect of the C2C program on participants' mental health outcomes and service-related programmatic outputs. The main research questions are

1. Do C2C program participants have increased access to and use of mental health services relative to comparison group members?
2. Do C2C participants show greater positive improvement in mental health, substance use and misuse, and functioning relative to comparison group members?
3. Do C2C program participants show improved educational attainment, housing stability, and employment outcomes after receiving C2C services relative to comparison group members assessed over the same time frame?

The primary inclusion criterion for the impact study is a positive screen for one or more of the following mental health conditions: depression, anxiety, PTSD, alcohol abuse, or drug abuse. The impact evaluation focuses on these conditions because these are the most common issues among the target populations, the CBOs have identified these as the most relevant for their specific target populations, and they are the conditions for which CBOs are screening clients as part of C2C. There are two key reasons that screening positive for a mental health condition is an inclusion criterion. First, this criterion is consistent with the focus of C2C; while the program has larger goals related to community well-being and system-level change, C2C's immediate focus is on increasing access to mental health care for those with or at high risk for a mental health condition. Screening positive for a mental health condition is evidence that the individual is in this high-risk group. Second, it is unlikely that individuals with very few or no mental health symptoms would exhibit any detectable change (i.e., measurable impact) in mental health symptoms or service utilization. Thus, the impact study focuses on individuals who have screened positive for one of the common mental health conditions above. Of note, the impact evaluation uses a low scoring threshold for determining study eligibility from the screeners in order to maximize the number of eligible individuals and to include participants with mild, moderate, and severe mental health symptoms, as is likely representative of the C2C participant population (as opposed to including only those with problems meeting a clinical threshold). The study eligibility criteria are shown in Table 2.2, along with published scoring criteria for each measure.

Table 2.2. Impact Evaluation Eligibility Criteria on Screening Measures

Screening Measure	Impact Evaluation Eligibility	Published Scoring Criteria	Reference
Patient Health Questionnaire–8 (PHQ-8)	Total score ≥5	0–4 = none to minimal depression 5–9 = mild depression 10–14 = moderate depression 15–19 = moderately severe depression 20–24 = severe depression	Kroenke et al., 2009
Generalized Anxiety Disorder–7 (GAD-7)	Total score ≥5	5 = mild anxiety 10 = moderate anxiety 15 = severe anxiety	Löwe et al., 2008; Spitzer et al., 2006
PTSD Checklist for DSM–5 (PCL-5)	Total score ≥28	≥33 = provisional PTSD diagnosis	Blevins et al., 2015
Alcohol Use Disorder Identification Test–10 (AUDIT-10)	Total score ≥8	≥ 8 = harmful or hazardous drinking ≥13 (women), ≥15 (men) = alcohol dependence	Babor et al., 1992; Berner et al., 2007
Drug Abuse Screening Test–10 (DAST-10)	Total score ≥1	0 = none 1–2 = low 3–5 = intermediate 6–8 = substantial 9–10 = severe	Yudko et al., 2007

The impact evaluation tests the extent to which C2C improves participants' access to mental health care and well-being on a variety of dimensions by comparing C2C clients with clients who receive similar services, but not C2C services, from similar local CBOs. The impact evaluation uses a quasiexperimental design, with longitudinal assessments administered at baseline, six months, and 12 months using a web-based data collection system. The quasiexperimental design allows for comparisons between the C2C intervention group and the comparison group without the requirement of random assignment. Comparison group participants were recruited from CBOs in New York City that serve similar populations (e.g., geographic location, race/ethnicity, primary language, age) and provide similar services (e.g., workforce development, youth development, homeless shelter, domestic violence shelter, immigrant-serving organization, early childhood) as C2C CBOs but are not implementing C2C or providing other mental health services.

Participant Enrollment

Study enrollment for the impact evaluation began in June 2017 and is expected to continue through March 2019. The primary inclusion criterion for the impact evaluation is meeting a minimum threshold on one or more of the eligibility screening measures for the common mental health conditions detailed above. All eligibility screeners are conducted in person. The baseline assessment is conducted after the eligibility screener and includes measures of quality of life, functioning, trauma history, stressful experiences, barriers to accessing mental health care, attitudes toward seeking mental health care, and mental health service utilization. The follow-up assessment includes the screening and baseline assessment measures in addition to questions about any services or supports received from CBO staff related to mood, thinking, or behavior. The baseline and follow-up assessments are conducted in person or via telephone. Both the eligibility screener and the baseline and follow-up assessments are administered in Spanish or English. Appendix A provides more details on the measures used for the eligibility screening, the baseline assessment, and the six- and 12-month follow-up assessments.

For the C2C CBOs, we worked closely with program staff to integrate the study data collection procedures into client work flow. Most CBOs follow the process depicted in Figure 2.1. First, CBO staff conduct the C2C screenings, offer clients the opportunity to participate in the C2C impact evaluation, and provide them with recruitment materials. Clients who are interested in participating in the study are referred by CBO staff to our collection staff, who obtain informed consent to participate in eligibility screening. If the CBO conducted their C2C screening using one or more of the five impact evaluation eligibility screening measures, CBO staff provide us with results from their C2C screenings to be used for study eligibility determination, so that clients need not repeat those measures for evaluation purposes. Data collection staff enter results from the C2C screening instruments into the web-based eligibility screener and administer any of the remaining impact evaluation screeners not already performed. If a client's scores on any of the screening measures deem them eligible to participate in the study, our staff advises the client that he or she is eligible to participate in the C2C impact evaluation and may be recruited into the study. If the client is interested in participating in the study, our staff obtain informed consent for the baseline assessment and administer the web-based baseline survey to the client. These procedures vary across organizations depending on their preferred workflow (e.g., CBO staff administer the study screening and then hand off eligible clients to our staff). C2C study participants receive a $20 gift card for completing the baseline assessment.

Figure 2.1. Data Collection Process at C2C CBOs

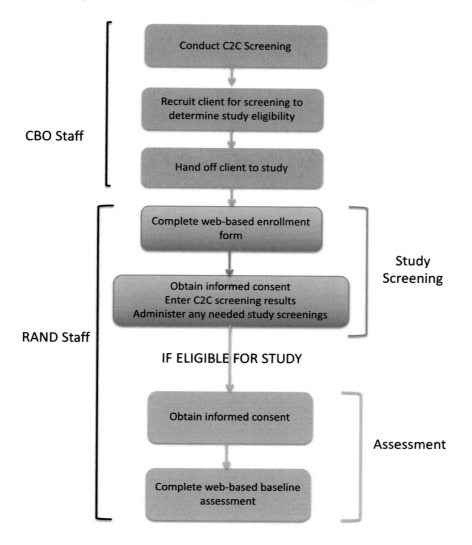

For the comparison CBOs, CBO staff support study recruitment (e.g., through recruitment events, inviting clients to the study during program intake, flyers), and our data collection staff complete the study screening and baseline assessment for those eligible for the study (Figure 2.2). Comparison group participants receive a $10 gift card for completing the eligibility screening and a $20 gift card for the baseline assessment. For both comparison and C2C participants, incentive gift cards at the six- and 12-month follow-ups are valued at $40 and $60, respectively.

Figure 2.2. Data Collection Process at Comparison CBOs

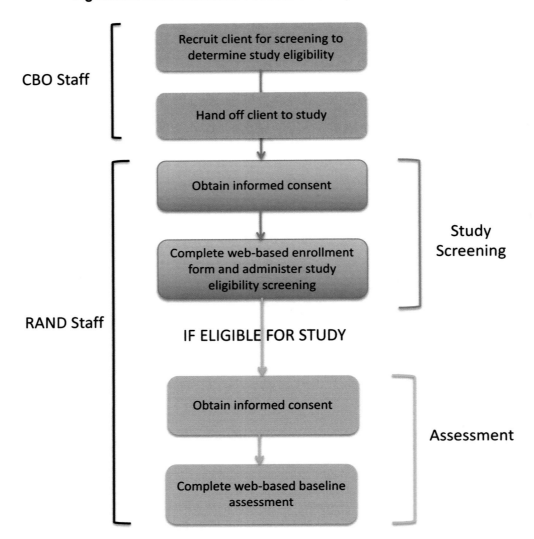

Data Collection

After eligibility screening, the data collection procedures are the same for those in the comparison and C2C groups. The baseline assessment includes the collection of contact information from study participants so that evaluators can maintain contact and locate them for their six-month follow-up assessment. Interim contact activities include sending postcards, emailing, texting, and calling study participants at specified intervals. We have defined a 2.5-month window during which we attempt to schedule and complete the six-month follow-up assessment. The window begins two weeks before the target date for the follow-up assessment and ends two months after that date. To schedule the six-month follow-up assessment, we use multiple methods (e.g., text, email, phone call) to locate the participant and schedule the survey in-person or over the phone. Data collection for follow-up assessments is expected to continue through March 2020.

The impact evaluation is conducting analyses of groups of CBOs (i.e., it will not examine findings at the individual CBO level), under the assumption that the interventions across C2C CBOs are similar to each other. Given this analytic assumption, it was not possible to include two organizations in the impact component of the evaluation. One CBO had contractual problems with its MHP that led to an extended delay to its implementation start; the other launched implementation with an intervention model that was substantially different from the other CBOs.

In Chapter 4 of this interim report, we provide a description of data collection progress so far, as well as baseline status for the intervention (C2C) portion of the sample of participants. Specifically, we describe the C2C sample's demographic characteristics, baseline symptom levels, barriers to mental health care access, readiness to engage in mental health care, and mental health care service use. All data come from the baseline client self-report survey.

Though not included in this interim report, final impact evaluation analyses will also include data from C2C CBOs that serve as indicators of C2C dosage. C2C dosage can help to determine whether participants who received more C2C services showed greater improvement over time compared with those who received less of the intervention. Data from New York City and New York state agencies will serve as indicators of health care use, justice system involvement, employment, and other outcomes. In the final analyses, the comparison group will be weighted to be demographically similar to the intervention group using propensity score weighting.

Cost Evaluation

It is too early to present data from the cost evaluation at this time. However, for descriptive purposes, we provide information about its goals and methods here. The cost evaluation has three goals: (1) to quantify the resources required to implement and maintain C2C, (2) to estimate the effect of C2C on medical spending and government expenditures, and (3) to estimate C2C's net savings from the perspectives of the city and state governments of New York and of the federal government. A more detailed description of the cost evaluation measures is provided in Appendix A.

To estimate the total cost of resources used in the C2C program, we will measure labor costs (e.g., salaries, wages, benefits), nonlabor costs (e.g., variable costs such as travel and supplies), CBO payments to MHPs and other vendors, and overhead costs. The primary data sources will include the quarterly CBO financial reports submitted to the Mayor's Fund, cost-related questions from the biannual cost surveys, the annual nonlabor expense report, and the annual compensation report. Up-front investments in fixed assets and the cost of planning or training needed to get the program started will also be measured. The resources used after the program matures, which may vary by CBO, will determine ongoing (or maintenance) costs. In the analysis, we will depreciate or amortize the upfront investment over time to ensure the costs are appropriately estimated.

To estimate the economic impact of C2C—the program's effect on medical spending and government expenditures—we will conduct an analysis of primary data from impact study participants and administrative data from government agencies. Data sources will include the baseline and follow-up impact study assessments, as well as New York City and New York State administrative data. Key estimates will include employment income and associated income taxes and the cost of medical (including behavioral health) care for C2C participants. Estimates will also approximate changes in government expenditures, such as unemployment benefits, cash/food assistance, housing subsidies, and justice system costs for these individuals.

To estimate potential net savings, we will combine the estimates of total cost and economic impact to determine whether the C2C program results in net savings. We anticipate that it may be difficult to detect individual-level savings associated with C2C within the 12-month study period. In other words, because of the study time frame, any savings may be underestimated in terms of savings.

Data Analyses

This section describes the qualitative and quantitative data analyses that we conducted for this interim report.

Qualitative Data

We used a mixed-method software environment (Dedoose) to conduct thematic analysis and identify recurring patterns in the interview data ("themes"). A team of four coders, all of whom participated in data collection (site visits), engaged in iterative rounds of data analysis to inform the development of a hierarchical code tree consisting of key themes. These coders held frequent coding reconciliation meetings to establish a robust shared sense of how the code tree represented the data and to ensure that coding was consistent. Analysis of qualitative data in this interim report reflects findings from the first wave of data collection only. More-detailed information on qualitative data analysis, including the final code tree, and results will be presented in the forthcoming final evaluation report in 2020.

Quantitative Data

Implementation Evaluation

We analyzed quantitative data from the staff survey and quarterly report using SAS version 9.4 and Excel. We conducted univariate analyses (e.g., means, percentages, counts) to describe implementation measures, including frequency and type of C2C training and coaching, delivery of C2C skills to clients, staff behaviors toward clients with mental health issues, and mental health knowledge and attitudes.

Impact Evaluation

We analyzed baseline client self-report survey data using the R statistical program. We conducted descriptive analyses to examine frequencies, means, and standard deviations of key baseline characteristics, including demographics, mental health symptoms, barriers to mental health care, and service utilization.

Cost Evaluation

Data for the cost evaluation are not presented at this time.

3. Interim Implementation Evaluation Findings

In this chapter, we provide an overview of variations in the implementation of C2C. We then describe early findings on implementation of specific components of C2C: CBO and MHP roles, training, supervision and coaching, staff readiness to deliver C2C, C2C service delivery, and perceived impact of C2C. The sections that follow summarize preliminary findings from years 1 and 2 of C2C implementation.

C2C Implementation Model Design

As described in Chapter 1, the C2C intervention employs a model of service delivery known as task shifting to increase access to mental health services by training lay CBO staff members (i.e., non–mental health specialists) to deliver mental health services to clients and facilitate referrals to more-intensive mental health treatment if needed. The C2C intervention requires that CBOs work collaboratively with MHPs to tailor the C2C intervention model to the needs of each organization's clients and staff members and ensure an optimal fit within the community setting.

At a minimum, CBOs are required to deliver training and follow-up support to CBO staff members in four core C2C skills: mental health screening, MHFA, MI, and psychoeducation. MHPs provided CBOs with expert input on the development and implementation of trainings, coaching and supervision programs, crisis management protocols, and referral practices. However, individual sites could choose which screening tools and psychoeducation content to implement. They could also decide when, where, and how the C2C skills were delivered in the context of existing programming. In addition, sites are not limited to implementing only the four core C2C skills; as their programs mature, they can build upon this framework, adding services and supports and adopting strategies that address the specific mental health needs of their client base and the broader communities they serve.

At program outset, CBOs and MHPs received guidance and technical assistance from the C2C Collaborative and McSilver Institute for Poverty Policy and Research at the New York University Silver School of Social Work (NYU McSilver) regarding required core implementation activities expected of each CBO-MHP pair. Based on this guidance, CBOs and MHPs worked collaboratively to develop a detailed operational plan document at the beginning of year 1; this document described plans for staffing, training, program implementation, MHP roles and responsibilities, and data collection. CBOs submitted their operational plans for multiple rounds of review to the C2C Collaborative, and they used feedback to iterate on the plans in close collaboration with technical assistance liaisons from the C2C Collaborative, RAND, and NYU McSilver. Webinars, email and phone communication, and in-person site visits were also used to identify and resolve potential issues with the plans.

Based on implementation strengths and challenges identified through program monitoring and technical assistance activities in year 1, the C2C Collaborative issued additional implementation guidance in May 2017. This updated guidance was designed to help CBOs and MHPs deepen the quality and scale of implementation by applying known best practices, clarifying implementation roles, and continuing to adapt the C2C model to specific CBO contexts. CBOs and MHPs were invited to share feedback on a draft guidance document in March 2017, and their input informed the document released in May 2017. The C2C Collaborative determined that many sites were experiencing challenges with expectations for psychoeducation delivery; determining which activities should not be handled by the CBO alone, but required MHP leadership; establishing robust coaching and supervision structures for CBO staff members who delivered C2C skills; and setting up care coordination processes. In response to these challenges, the revised implementation guidance issued in May 2017 included the following clarifications:

- It required that CBOs implement a curriculum-based and evidence-informed psychoeducation program that is matched to observed or self-reported need(s) of CBO participants.
- It clarified MHP roles with regard to protocol development, coaching and supervision, and fidelity monitoring.
- It established a requirement of quarterly coaching/supervision for staff trained in any of the C2C skills and required the use of relevant best practices, such as direct practice observation, in coaching and supervision.
- It clarified that, at least once per quarter, MHP and CBO staff who participate in the screening, referral, and care coordination process must take part in an interdisciplinary case review.

Following the issuance of this guidance, CBOs and MHPs revised their operational plans to accommodate the stated requirements. Figure 3.1 describes these and the other year 1 and 2 implementation activities that will be discussed in this chapter.

Figure 3.1. Key Implementation Events for CBOs, Years 1–2

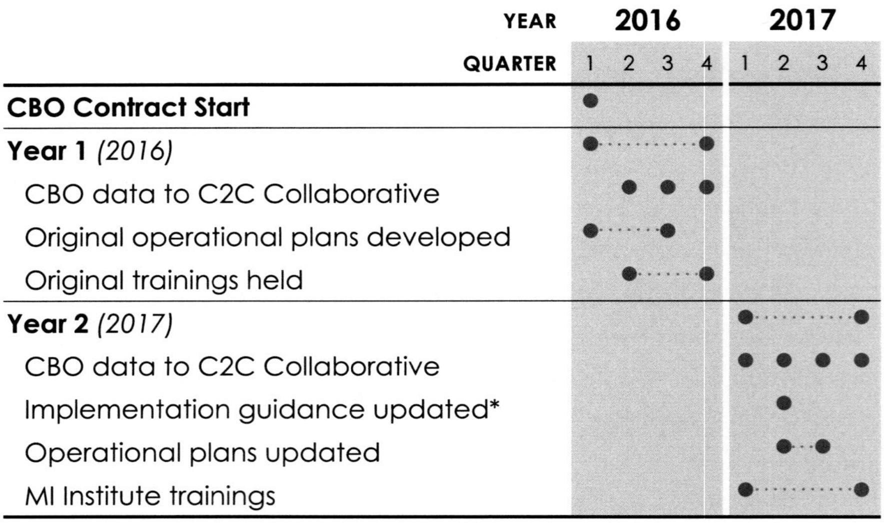

	2016 Q1	Q2	Q3	Q4	2017 Q1	Q2	Q3	Q4
CBO Contract Start	●							
Year 1 *(2016)*	●·········●							
CBO data to C2C Collaborative		●	●	●				
Original operational plans developed	●········●							
Original trainings held		●·······●						
Year 2 *(2017)*					●·········●			
CBO data to C2C Collaborative					●	●	●	●
Implementation guidance updated*						●		
Operational plans updated						●··●		
MI Institute trainings					●·········●			

*Implementation guidance included clarifications on delivery of curriculum-based psychoeducation, minimum screening requirements, minimum coaching and supervision requirements, care coordination, and soliciting client and staff feedback on program delivery.

In addition to the original and updated operational plan guidance, sites also participate in ongoing program monitoring, technical assistance, and learning network activities. During the first two program years, offerings included multiple webinars and meetings hosted by the C2C Collaborative to describe expectations and best practices on topics, including, but not limited to, continuous QI, data collection and reporting procedures, and supervision practices (e.g., use of reflective supervision).

Aarons et al. (2011) presented a conceptual model for implementation of evidence-based practices that can serve as a helpful guide in contextualizing C2C implementation thus far. According to that model, the first phase of implementation is "Exploration," during which organizations increase awareness of some need, challenge, or approach that could be improved or addressed. The next phase is "Adoption Decision/Preparation," during which organizations plan and prepare for implementation, including which approaches to take and how they will implement their selected intervention(s). The third phase is "Active Implementation" of the intervention, and the fourth and final phase is "Sustainment." At the time of primary data collection (i.e., key informant interviews and staff survey in summer 2017) in year 2, organizations were in the Adoption Decision/Preparation phase and early stages of Active Implementation. All organizations had begun conducting C2C training and delivering some C2C skills to clients, but sites varied considerably with respect to timelines for initiating specific activities (e.g., training for specific skills, such as MI; continuous coaching and supervision). In addition, at the time of primary data collection, many organizations were in the process of modifying aspects of their operational plans (e.g., for psychoeducation training) in response to the changes in implementation guidance described above. Due to this variability in implementation, we present aggregate findings and common themes across organizations rather than comparing and contrasting individual sites or characterizing implementation progress by organization.

C2C Implementation Model Variations

Consistent with C2C flexibility to tailor the model according to the CBO context and populations served, implementation models for C2C varied considerably across organizations. Organizations differed in their intended degree of task shifting, as defined by the number and types of staff members that delivered each of the four core C2C skills. Most organizations trained a wide variety of staff members in MHFA, such as administrative staff and security management, for the purpose of increasing mental health awareness broadly within the organization. However, they reserved training in other supports (screening, psychoeducation, MI) for a smaller group of client-facing staff members. Other CBOs trained different types of staff members in different supports based on typical client case flow. For example, at some sites, training in screening was provided only to those individuals who conducted client intakes (when initial screening occurred), whereas psychoeducation training was provided only to staff members who led classes or workshops that involved psychoeducation curricula. Some CBOs relied primarily on one or two staff members with professional training in a mental health-related field (e.g., licensed clinical social workers) to deliver the majority of C2C skills to clients in the early stages of the implementation process (e.g., as a means of "pilot testing" the C2C program), with plans to expand training to additional staff members over time. Still others took the approach of training only a core group of direct service or client-facing staff members in all four supports.

The novelty and flexibility of the C2C program was viewed by many interviewees as both an exciting opportunity to innovate and meet the needs of clients and staff members and as a challenge. Some CBO leaders were enthusiastic about the prospect of breaking new ground to address client needs:

> I realize we're on the ground floor of this project and everyone is figuring it out as we go along. That carries great opportunity—and great frustration—so I'm kind of honored to be in on this . . . . What a great opportunity to figure it out and hopefully create a national model.

Communication from the C2C Collaborative, such as ongoing technical assistance, solicitation of CBO and MHP feedback through regular correspondence, surveys to assess organizations' needs and experiences with C2C, and written guidance (i.e., implementation guidance documents) on recommendations for implementing C2C, were seen as helpful and responsive to such concerns during the early stages of the implementation process. However, as stated by one CBO leader, "just keeping up with all those constant and ongoing changes [was] a challenge" during the first year of implementation. The gradual approach to rolling out the C2C program in the first year, along with the freedom to adapt the program to meet unique needs of different organizations, were nonetheless seen as reducing burden and stress on CBO staff members:

> For implementation, I appreciated the fact that it wasn't a big onslaught. Like "You're going to learn all of this right away." I appreciated the fact that it was rolled out gradually and they allowed us flexibility, and there seems to be recognition that not every sector is the same and therefore there appears to be a lot of room to work this out as we go. And that it's being rolled out over time has been a wise move, I think.

CBO and MHP Roles

The roles of CBOs and MHPs in the C2C model were designed so that CBOs could benefit from the mental health expertise of MHPs and MHPs could learn from CBOs about client context, understand how to expand mental health service capacity through teaching, and develop stronger ties to surrounding communities. MHPs were required to contribute to a range of activities, including receiving referrals and facilitating access to clinical care, training and supervising CBO staff, consulting in difficult cases, consulting on program design and implementation decisions, and delivering C2C mental health skills to CBO clients. MHPs were also expected to help CBOs tailor the C2C model to each organization and to provide input on how to design and implement the C2C mental health skills in each setting.

To accommodate setting-specific differences, the C2C model allowed for flexibility in designating specific responsibilities to CBO and MHP staff members. All MHPs contributed to development and implementation of staff training activities, as well as development or review of crisis management and client mental health referral protocols. However, the extent and nature of MHP involvement in implementing components of the C2C program (e.g., supervision/coaching, delivering C2C mental health skills, referral processes) varied considerably across organizations. Based on interviews and reviews of CBO operational plans, such differences may be attributable to variations in CBO and MHP characteristics, including

- size and number of CBO locations
- type of programming, work flow, and client "case flow" at the CBO
- on-site presence of the MHP
- relationship between the CBO and MHP (e.g., affiliate organization versus external partner)
- capacity and capabilities of MHPs to design and implement training and supervision in each C2C mental health support
- capacity and capabilities of CBOs to carry out activities requiring specialized mental health knowledge and skills.

For example, a number of CBOs employed one or more staff members with professional training in a mental health–related field (e.g., counselors, clinical social workers, psychologists) prior to C2C. These sites were often able to leverage the experience of CBO staff members to help implement training and supervision activities. In contrast, sites with few or no staff members with professional training in a mental health–related field tended to rely more heavily on the MHP for training and oversight in delivery of the C2C skills. Other CBOs had MHPs that were located on the premises of main CBO site or worked within the same parent organization but were located at different sites. In such cases, some CBOs had an existing level of interaction and communication with the MHP prior to C2C, but others did not.

MHP Presence at CBO Sites

Some implementation models included a staff member who was affiliated with both the MHP and CBO, occupying substantive roles at both organizations (e.g., providing clinical services at the MHP and coordinating C2C activities at the CBO). Interviewees who experienced this model shared that having a dually affiliated staff person was helpful in "uniting" CBO and MHP program activities and streamlining communication between organizations. For example, when asked to describe the dually affiliated C2C coordinator, one CBO staff member said:

> Basically, she is a bridge. She is the bridge between [the CBO] and the clinic. I think also having her physically in [the CBO], she sees families and the processes of enrollment and sees our engagement and interactions and she works very much as a liaison between [the MHP] and [the CBO]. She's been phenomenal in her role.

Other implementation models specified having an MHP staff member on-site at the CBO for a certain number of hours each week. The time spent on-site at the CBO and the nature of the MHP staff's tasks while onsite varied; some were on-site primarily for the provision of training and coaching or supervision of CBO staff, while others made themselves available to receive "warm handoff" referrals and to provided client services on-site. (See also *Client Referrals* section below.)

The on-site presence of MHP staff was viewed as particularly helpful in increasing CBO staff and client familiarity with MHP staff members. MHP staff who provided client services at the CBO were seen as reducing barriers to referral follow-through, as well as increasing accessibility of more-intensive mental health services for clients experiencing mental health difficulties. One CBO staff member stated:

> I think we are looking forward to having someone on-site. It is not only counseling that [clients] don't always follow through with, sometimes it is even their case management meetings that they don't follow through with and they have a lot on their plate, so bringing someone [from the MHP] on-site should help make it [mental health services] more accessible.

Efforts to integrate MHPs into the CBO environment were also viewed as beneficial in enhancing clients' familiarity and reducing discomfort with MHPs, which has implications for facilitating referrals to MHPs. For example, staff cited clients' discomfort sharing personal and private information with people they do not know well, which historically has created barriers for CBO staff during the referral process. A CBO staff member shared a referral experience:

> Clients have built a relationship with you—clients have shared their story with you and they don't want to now go to another person to share the same story all over again. At the beginning, it is very hard, and it takes a lot of work to convince them that this other person will help them and that they can trust that person as much as they have trusted me.

In some instances, MHPs—who were expected to provide support and guidance to CBOs on tailoring the C2C model for each site—experienced struggles in meeting the technical assistance needs of CBOs. As noted by one MHP leader:

> It felt like we were starting from scratch . . . . [It was unclear] what exactly to train the staff on in terms of psychoeducation, and how we were going to supervise. There was so much openness to it, and that made it hard.

Differences between expected and actual capacity of MHPs to direct training decisions and provide training and coaching for all of the core C2C skills presented some difficulties in the early stages of the implementation process. The majority of MHPs found designing and enacting implementation of MI, in particular, to be quite challenging, especially for MHPs with limited expertise in the skill (see *Training* section below). For example, one MHP leader reported:

> We didn't realize how hard it was to actually train and supervise MI so that set us back and finding someone with those skills was really hard. People are not as available as we thought they would be, and it also cost more than we thought to offer these trainings.

Although such difficulties were initially a source of frustration, many MHPs also valued the opportunity to expand their clinical and supervisory skill sets by participating in more-intensive MI training provided by the Mayor's Fund (see *Training* section).

CBO and MHP Relationships

As noted above, CBOs structured their relationships with MHPs in various ways, and all interviewed CBO and MHP leads viewed these relationships as critical to the success of C2C. Yet many interviewees shared that they experienced some difficulties in developing a strong collaborative relationship early on because of communication challenges, CBO lack of familiarity with MHP services and protocol, and MHP lack of knowledge about CBO clients and services. In some instances, such initial challenges were anticipated, as most CBOs and MHPs had not previously collaborated on projects of similar magnitude and had limited understanding of one another's organizations prior to the launch of the C2C program. For example, some interviewees acknowledged that CBOs and MHP differed regarding institutional cultures, norms, and job expectations. One MHP leader said of the early challenges of working together:

> How to work with the culture of this organization [CBO] and not impact or overwhelm the [CBO] staff so much with a cultural change. And sometimes

34

some of the [CBO] staff wouldn't want to ask some of the questions in the screening because they were afraid of all that may come up. And learning how much time they have to give to this; it seems like they enjoy being part of this—but [the C2C program] is asking if they can do this and still cover everything else and also learning how to deal with their own emotions as they are conducting these screenings.

Similarly, MHP interviewees noted that navigating differences in organizational cultures was an early challenge to developing effective working relationships with CBOs. For example:

My idea of this program is almost to change the culture, and that is a challenge logistically. There are plenty of meetings and constant back and forth. Other natural challenges are that some people are hesitant to use this, so staff buy-in can be challenging. Infusing mental health into everything can seem overwhelming; I think that is one of the challenges to be expected.

CBO leaders echoed these sentiments regarding differences in organizational cultures. One CBO leader reported:

We're very different systems. And [our MHP] is this huge institution and we're very small, so we do think a little differently. So just getting that understanding and working on it. It took a little bit in the beginning, but now we're able to figure out how each system works.

Jointly navigating these challenges required close collaboration between organizational leaders and staff members. Efforts by CBO and MHP staff to learn about each other's organizations were seen as helpful in building a stronger program model, even for CBOs and MHPs under the same parent organization. As noted by one CBO lead, whose MHP was part of the same parent organization:

From the MHP side, they really like getting to know more about [the CBO] and our clients, so it has provided them more context on our clients too, whereas before the C2C program, there wasn't as much of an interface between [the MHP] and our agency.

Frequent and open lines of communication between CBOs and MHPs (e.g., regularly scheduled and ad hoc phone meetings; email exchanges; regular in-person meetings) were said to be helpful in building more effective relationships, collaboratively working toward implementation goals, and navigating challenges that arose early in the implementation process. One MHP leader described this type of communication:

[We have] open communication and the same goals. We communicate very well in what we need, whenever there is a problem, we don't wait until an official meeting, we pick up the phone and bring it up. CBO leadership and MHP leadership have monthly meetings—we discuss new ideas, what else we need to establish, etc.

In addition, efforts to familiarize CBO staff members with MHP staff by attending joint meetings and holding "meet and greet" events were seen as helpful for improving communication, fostering a better understanding among CBO staff of MHP culture, and ensuring positive working relationships between staff at both organizations. C2C coordinators also played a critical role in facilitating effective communication between CBOs and MHPs:

> When we [MHP] have a meeting [with CBO], the C2C coordinator always has a very detailed agenda for us which I appreciate, and she is also always conscious of the time so that we don't get side tracked and so all of that helps tremendously.

Another CBO leader described the importance of regular contact in maintaining a strong CBO-MHP collaboration:

> [The MHP] is very responsive to our team and our staff overall, he makes himself very available to provide counseling, he comes in consistently every Thursday and he leads our clinical monthly meetings, so that has been a great relationship.

Mutual agreement on the respective roles and responsibilities of CBOs and MHPs was also viewed as a critical component of successful implementation of the C2C program. As reported by one MHP leader:

> With us, each person has a very specific role, and this is my role. . . . I think for me and them it was a matter of just trying to understand how we can meet each other in the middle and figure out how we can move forward without me assuming that "you're doing this" or you assuming that "I'm doing this" and somebody dropping the ball.

Training

CBOs and MHPs worked collaboratively to design training protocols for each of the four C2C skills. While trainings for MHFA were preselected, other training protocols had to be chosen (e.g., for psychoeducation curricula) or developed (e.g., protocols for administering screenings) by CBOs and MHPs, and then implemented. Although MHPs were expected to assist in development and implementation of training plans, not all MHPs had the capacity to train in the four core modalities at the outset. CBOs and MHPs included training plans for each skill in their operational plans in year 1, and updated as needed in year 2, although the specificity of plans varied considerably across organizations. Technical assistance liaisons from the C2C Collaborative provided extensive input to some CBOs on how to select a curriculum-based psychoeducation program based on client needs.

Within-Organization Trainings

All CBOs used MHP staff members to implement training in the C2C skills, but specific training plans varied considerably across organizations. In most cases, both CBO and MHP staff members led some C2C training activities, though organizations typically arranged for the MHP to administer all C2C trainings during the early implementation period. All CBOs leveraged MHP leaders to help design training protocols for screening. As noted above, organizations were required to incorporate screening tools for depression, anxiety, and substance use, but were able to include other screening materials based upon perceived needs of their client populations. For example, several sites also incorporated screenings for trauma history and/or PTSD. MHPs helped CBOs select screening tools and develop and implement site-specific training materials for CBO staff, which detailed best practices for introducing, administering, and discussing results with clients.

CBOs received guidance from their MHPs and technical assistance liaisons on how to identify the specific needs of their participants and select psychoeducation programs that addressed behavioral health topics aligned with these needs. MHPs worked with CBOs to select and implement trainings in evidence-based psychoeducation curricula. In some instances, both MHPs and CBOs learned and implemented a "new" program together; in other cases, the MHP trained the CBO staff in a program in which they already had expertise; in still others, CBOs and MHPs sought training from curriculum developers. Many CBOs found that off-the-shelf trainings in psychoeducation curricula required substantial tailoring to match the needs and context of their client populations, and they worked closely with their MHPs and technical assistance liaisons to make these changes. Psychoeducation curriculum content areas included mindfulness-based stress reduction, coping with trauma and PTSD, substance abuse and relapse prevention, positive parenting behaviors, and developing resiliency, self-care, and positive coping skills. Most trainings in delivery of psychoeducation curricula were implemented after the May 2017 change in implementation guidance for psychoeducation (see Figure 3.1). MHPs also delivered trainings in MI and MHFA in some organizations, although external trainings were made available to all CBOs for these two mental health supports (see *External Trainings* below), and many CBOs utilized these external resources in place of or in addition to MHP-led trainings.

External Trainings

CBO/MHP staff across all C2C organizations were offered externally led trainings in MHFA and MI. Unlike within-organization trainings, content was not tailored to each CBO. MHFA trainings followed a standard curriculum (more below); the MI curriculum was developed specifically for C2C providers, but not for individual organizations within C2C. These external trainings helped supplement MHP-led trainings and were seen as particularly helpful in instances where MHPs did not have initial capacity to provide training and supervision in these skills. Beyond these externally coordinated trainings, CBOs have the option to use C2C funds to hire external consultants or trainers to supplement MHP expertise, where needed. Some CBOs who were not able to participate in the centralized MI trainings developed for the C2C network, for example, chose to hire MI trainers who provided on-site training and coaching to CBO staff. Below, we provide additional information on the centralized MHFA and MI trainings made available to the C2C network.

Mental Health First Aid Trainings

Early in C2C implementation, MHFA trainings were provided at no cost to C2C CBO staff. The MHFA training was sponsored by the city-wide ThriveNYC initiative, which aims to train 250,000 New Yorkers in MHFA (New York City Department of Health and Mental Hygiene, 2018). Trainings took place at various locations throughout the city, and were made available in English and Spanish, with other languages available upon request. MHFA training uses a standardized, evidence-based curriculum. These one-day trainings were eight hours long, and each course was delivered by certified MHFA trainers who had undergone a standardized training and certification (Mental Health First Aid USA, 2012, 2018). Additional "train-the-trainer" sessions were made available to CBO and MHP staff; participating staff were certified as MHFA trainers and were then available for ongoing in-house assistance and training for CBO staff.

Motivational Interviewing Training

In summer 2016, the C2C Collaborative conducted a survey of MHPs to assess their readiness to train and supervise CBO staff in MI, psychoeducation, and screening. Eleven of the 15 MHPs responded to this survey, and findings indicated that many MHPs had limited experience and subject-matter expertise in providing training and supervision in at least one type of C2C support. This was particularly evident for MI, for which only three organizations employed providers with intermediate to advanced MI skills. Based on this gap, the Mayor's Fund contracted with an external training and technical assistance provider to help build capacity of both MHPs and CBOs in implementing MI training and supervision for the C2C program.

The C2C MI Institute was made available to staff members of participating CBOs and MHPs at no additional cost to CBOs. The program was designed to train and support CBO and MHP staff and leadership in MI, emphasizing a collaborative, nondirective, and nonjudgmental approach to discussing behavior change and enhancing client motivation to change through the use of specific skills (Miller and Rollnick, 2008, 2013). Distinct tracks were available for practitioners, supervisors, trainers, and organizational leads. Training occurred between December 2016 and December 2017.

- The *practitioner track* was open to CBO and MHP client-facing staff who desired training in MI. Practitioners were offered a two-day introductory training, monthly learning groups (two hours per month for eight months), web-based MI skill modules (ten minutes per week and additional practice time), and two fidelity assessment sessions that used Motivational Interviewing Treatment Integrity (MITI) coding (Moyers et al., 2005) and included written feedback on fidelity.
- The *supervisor track* was open to CBO and MHP staff who demonstrated MI proficiency through MITI coding. It included advanced MI skills training and specialized training to provide MI coaching and supervision. It included all elements of the *practitioner track* with additional components: a one-day advanced practice training and ongoing monthly supervisor learning groups (two hours per month for eight months). Additionally,

supervisor track participants who demonstrated a higher level of MI competence through MITI coding were invited to participate in a two-day intensive train-the-trainer workshop.

- The *implementation support track* was available to CBO leadership and was designed to help with the development of sustainable MI implementation in their respective CBO (e.g., promoting staff buy-in, incorporating MI into the organization's culture and practices). MHP leaders also had the opportunity to engage in the implementation support track. Leaders participating in the implementation support track participated in a four-hour implementation workshop and were invited to participate in four group implementation support calls facilitated by an MI expert.

In total, all 15 CBOs and 11 MHPs utilized the MI Institute, although participation levels varied by organization. Seventy-eight staff were trained in the practitioner track, and 49 were trained in the supervisor track. Additionally, 15 supervisor track participants completed a train-the-trainer workshop. All training sessions were led by members of the Motivational Interviewing Network of Trainers (MINT) (Motivational Interviewing Network of Trainers, 2017). Sessions consisted of didactic and practice-based components and incorporated substantial real-play and ongoing coaching to support staff skills development and self-efficacy to deliver the MI support.

After using the MI Institute, several CBOs have developed in-house MI training and support, including internal MI trainings based on the Institute materials and voluntary MI practice groups. In addition, eight CBOs/MHPs voluntarily submitted MI implementation plans for review by the MINT trainers who facilitated the MI Institute. In response to challenges identified in those plans, MINT trainers also developed an MI implementation guide for the C2C network. Finally, online resources (e.g., presentation slides, training and coaching exercises, fidelity tools) were made available by the MI Institute to all C2C organizations to support ongoing training and implementation efforts.

Participation in C2C Trainings

A total of 1,225 CBO staff members (including 1,029 direct service staff members and 196 supervisors) were trained in C2C skills between March 2016 and March 2018, including internal and external trainings. Total participation in trainings surpassed overall CBO targets of 669 staff trained in year 1 (126-percent participation) and 241 staff trained in year 2 (148-percent participation). Individual CBO training targets varied considerably, ranging from seven to 98 in year 1 (mean = 45; median = 34), and from five to 60 in year 2 (mean = 16; median = 10).

Figure 3.2 shows the total number of staff members trained in any of the C2C skills over time (by quarter). As expected, the increase in number of CBO staff members trained was highest during the first year of implementation and slowed in year 2 after sites had largely established and implemented trainings in each of the four core C2C skills. Total numbers of staff members trained varied across CBOs, from 20 staff members to more than 270 staff members in a given organization (mean = 82; median = 55). Fourteen out of 15 CBOs met or surpassed their total training targets for the first two years. By March 2018, 181 direct service staff and 64 supervisors were trained in all four core C2C skills.

Figure 3.2. Cumulative Number of Staff Trained in C2C Skills

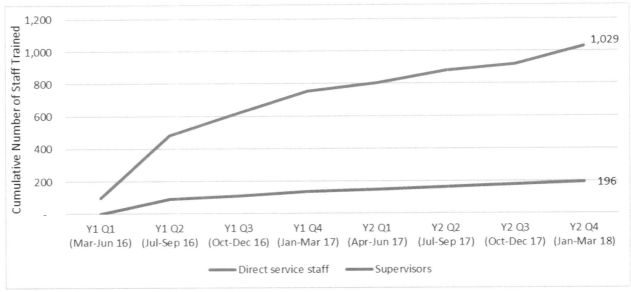

SOURCE: Data from quarterly CBO reports provided to RAND staff, 2016–2018.

Figure 3.3 shows the total number of staff trained in each C2C skill over time. Most organizations prioritized training in MHFA early in the implementation process, capitalizing on the availability of free external MHFA trainings (through ThriveNYC). MHFA was typically the first type of C2C support in which CBO staff members were trained, largely because it was viewed as providing a useful introduction to behavioral health issues for staff members without formal education in a behavioral health–related field. In addition, because trainings were external and content was standardized, organizations were able to initiate MHFA trainings earlier in the implementation process compared with trainings in other core skills, which typically required time to develop and tailor to setting-specific needs. As noted by one CBO leader, MHFA trainings were seen as being "very concrete" and "very helpful for staff that doesn't have [a] clinical background."

Figure 3.3. Number of Staff Trained, by Year and C2C Skills

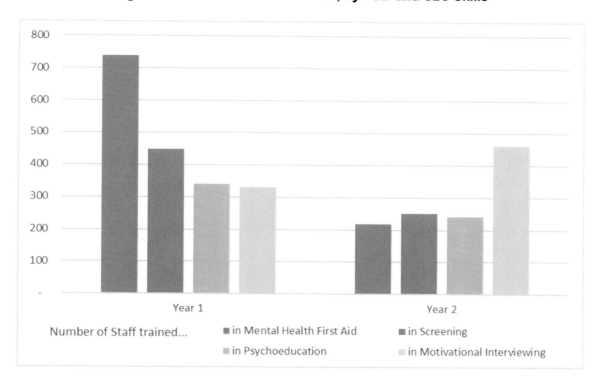

SOURCE: Data from quarterly CBO reports provided to RAND staff, 2016–2018.
NOTE: Individual staff may have been trained in more than one modality per quarter.

Between March 2016 and March 2018, CBOs and MHPs spent a total of 1,407 hours delivering trainings in core C2C skills to CBO staff, with about two-thirds of the training hours provided by MHPs. Figure 3.4 shows number of training hours administered for each C2C support by both CBO and MHP trainers. CBOs and MHPs devoted the first quarter of the implementation period to developing and refining training plans and began delivering trainings in the second quarter of year 1. The number of training hours delivered by the MHP was greatest in the early stages of the implementation process, when initial C2C trainings were delivered to staff. Both MHP- and CBO-provided training hours then dropped over time, as the emphasis switched to training newer hires and coaching and supervision activities for staff who had already received initial training. The lowest quarter for training hours coincides with the time when CBOs and MHPs were revising implementation plans based on revised implementation guidance (as described in Chapter 1) and shifting focus toward continuous coaching for already-trained staff. One exception in the downward trend is a large increase in the number of training hours provided for MI in year 2, quarter 4. One possible reason for this spike is that CBO and MHP staff who completed the supervisor track of the externally provided MI training in December 2017 then began implementing MI trainings at their own organizations, starting in January 2018.

Figure 3.4. Number of Training Hours Provided by MHP and CBO

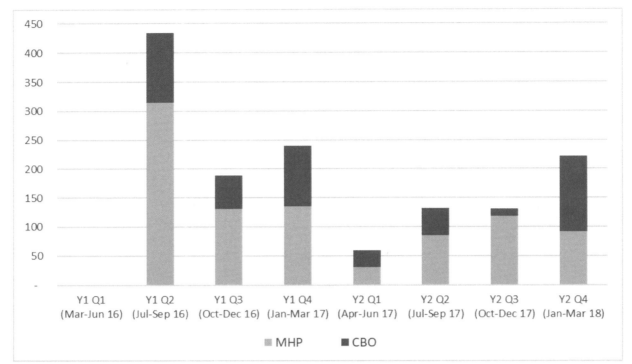

SOURCE: Data from quarterly CBO reports provided to RAND staff, 2016–2018.

As described in the "Implementation Model Variations" section above, there was considerable variability in the types of staff members trained in each of the four core C2C skills. For example, some organizations prioritized capacity for multiple types of staff members (e.g., social workers, administrative staff, educators, leadership) to deliver all types of C2C skills to clients. Other organizations only trained a subset of staff members—often social workers or other individuals with professional training in mental health-related fields—in specific C2C skills, such as psychoeducation and screening. CBO quarterly report data indicated that, on average across all quarters, approximately 12 percent of trainees received training in all four C2C skills.

This variability was also reflected in staff survey data, as shown in Figure 3.5. Consistent with many CBOs' implementation plans to stagger trainings, a majority of staff (87 percent) who completed the survey in summer 2017 (early in year 2) reported having received training in MHFA, whereas fewer had received training in the other C2C skills. Less than half (49 percent) of respondents reported receiving training in psychoeducation, although it is important to note that data were collected shortly after the distribution of updated implementation guidance for psychoeducation; therefore, many organizations had yet to implement training in curriculum-based psychoeducation at this stage.

Figure 3.5. Percentage of Staff Who Received Training in C2C Skills

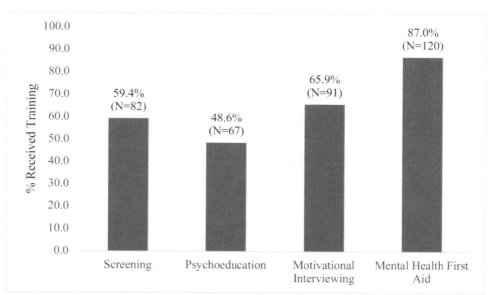

SOURCE: Data provided through annual survey of CBO staff, 2017.

Staff also varied with respect to the total number of C2C mental health supports in which they were trained as of summer 2017. As shown in Figure 3.6, nearly one-third (31 percent) of staff survey respondents indicated having been trained in the four core C2C mental health skills. Approximately one-quarter of staff members (27 percent) had received training in only one skill. Of individuals who only received training in one skill, most reported receiving training in MHFA only; these individuals accounted for 26 percent of all respondents. The most common training combinations were MHFA and MI (11 percent of respondents); screening, MHFA, and MI (10 percent of respondents); and screening, psychoeducation, and MHFA (6 percent of respondents). Of note, staff survey data represent a snapshot of staff experiences among those staff who had been trained in at least one C2C support as of summer 2017. Completion of the staff survey was voluntary, and not all staff offered the survey completed it. As such, survey findings do not include the experience of all staff trained by the end of year 2 ($n = 1,225$) and do not reflect developments in training in the latter half of year 2.

Figure 3.6. Proportion of Staff Reporting Number of C2C Support Training Types

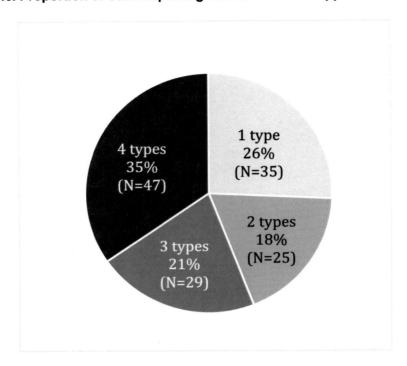

SOURCE: Data provided through annual survey of CBO staff, 2017.

Barriers and Facilitators to C2C Trainings

Turnover was viewed as a long-standing problem at several organizations although it was *not* seen as a problem that was brought on or exacerbated by the C2C program. In the staff survey, over 40 percent of respondents agreed or strongly agreed with the statement "Frequent staff turnover is a problem for this program." Some CBO personnel viewed staff turnover as a significant challenge for the implementation of C2C because C2C requires both initial and ongoing training. For example, as one CBO leader noted, "we trained over 100 staff last year, but we have a lot of staff turnover, so it feels like we are training all over again." This constant retraining of staff members was perceived to have slowed down the initial implementation of C2C because more effort than anticipated was needed to coordinate and implement trainings during the first year of implementation (i.e., in order to ensure that new hires were equipped to fulfill organizational expectations for C2C positions). Other organizations experienced relatively low turnover in C2C positions, but still noted that synthesizing and implementing all the new learning coming out of trainings was not a rapid process. As described by one interviewee:

> When you have new staff learning a new model and trying to implement a new model and trying to create a new partnership—in my mind, you're not going to see the results you want to see in year 1 under those conditions.

Both CBO and MHP leaders and staff members mentioned that the lack of knowledge about each other's services created barriers to implementing C2C trainings. When CBO staff had concerns surrounding the fit between C2C skills and their clients, some of them felt that they did not get adequate resolution of these concerns from MHPs and/or perceived that MHPs interpreted their concerns as resistance to delivering C2C skills. One CBO staff member shared an experience with an MHP trainer:

> I think our first trainer didn't have the background [for this CBO], so the expectations of how [the trainer] thought we could use [C2C skills] was not realistic. So, during the training, we brought up some of these challenges and they took that as us not wanting to do it, but that wasn't it.

In addition, some MHPs felt it was difficult to respond to challenges surrounding initial roll-out of C2C trainings because they were not members of the CBOs and did not have preexisting relationships with CBO staff. For example, one MHP leader said:

> I think it's difficult because as the MHP, I'm in the supervisory role on the clinical side but not for staff within [the CBO]. I don't have a voice [in how] things get done at the [the CBO]. I don't have authority to get staff to come to trainings. I have to be careful not to step on anyone's toes.

Similarly, MHP staff members also reported challenges related to limited knowledge of CBO organizational structure and policies, especially with regard to where and how to incorporate supervision of the C2C skills. One MHP leader described the challenge as:

> Knowing how [the CBO] works as far as staff supervision. Do they do case conferences? Where can we fit in? How are we describing C2C to the clients?

NYU McSilver attempted to mitigate some of these difficulties by strongly encouraging MHP participation in monthly technical assistance calls (and, occasionally, on-site provision of technical assistance) to guide CBO-MHP pairs through a facilitated discussion of training and organizational culture challenges. NYU McSilver also used monthly calls to share successful efforts from other CBO-MHP pairs navigating similar challenges, such as CBO tours of the an MHP; MHP shadowing of CBO staff; and "meet and greets," during which CBO and MHP staff could get to know each other better in a setting that was not related to training or supervision. Working through these early challenges appeared to improve communication. For example, the MHP leader quoted above also noted that "Actively coming and asking questions is working things out—it's getting better."

Feedback from interviews with CBO leaders indicated that efforts to openly address staff concerns during trainings helped ease some of the initial discomfort among CBO staff. One CBO leader shared:

> We are also very clear on the training that if they don't have clinical background they are not expected to have to calm clients down all on their own. We let them know that this is just to help them understand how to better deal with the clients and be more comfortable, having some tools accessible to them, but they know that they still have supervisors that can lead how they respond.

Similarly, MHP efforts to understand CBO staff and client needs—and to tailor C2C trainings for a nonclinical audience—helped to make training successful. For example, a CBO staff member shared an experience with MHP trainers:

> [I was] pleasantly surprised by C2C trainings and working with trainers. [The trainers] were very engaging and they understood our work and the potential staff resistance very well. They were able to roll out steps in [a] very manageable way.

Finally, CBO and MHP leaders highlighted the importance of taking staff feedback into account and using this information to augment C2C training; this was seen as critical for facilitating staff buy-in to C2C training, and for the C2C program more generally. One MHP leader said:

> I would definitely say that [staff buy-in] was one of the earlier challenges . . . . Staff have so much to do outside of C2C, so implementing it is kind of "another thing to do." So that's why the approach is to meet them where they are and identify how they want to use it and grow from there—and then hopefully buy-in will increase.

Staff Perceptions of Trainings

Overall, staff reported high rates of satisfaction with C2C training. In the survey of staff who participated in C2C trainings, around two-thirds (68 percent) of respondents agreed with the statement "I am satisfied with the training I have received in C2C mental health modalities." However, approximately one in three staff respondents did not agree with this statement, indicating that a substantial minority of trainees were not fully satisfied with some of their training experiences as of summer 2017. During key informant interviews, staff also generally reported high satisfaction with training. Interviewees commented on specific factors that helped to make trainings effective and useful. For example, several interviewees highlighted the importance of incorporating specific strategies like role plays. Others noted that efforts to tailor trainings to the needs of staff member and client population (e.g., by incorporating relevant examples) were particularly helpful in making the training applicable for participants. For example, one CBO leader said:

> He [MHP trainer] was so incredible and he met us where we're at regardless of our background, like he was learning from us as well as us learning from him. He also asked [CBO staff] for real situations they've encountered, which made it more applicable. It was great, and we're going to do part two soon.

Another CBO lead noted:

> As far as psychoeducation, I knew what it was but didn't have an expectation of what the training would look like. But as far as the feedback that we got from staff of what they thought of it and seeing the engagement and conversations during the training, I have to say that it worked for us. [MHP staff] did a great job of tailoring the training to our population.

Some interviewees specifically highlighted their positive experiences with the C2C MI Institute, emphasizing the benefits of having regular practice groups and follow-up support. One CBO leader shared:

> I think the continuity of the training—the recurrence of the trainings has really stood out to me because something very common is to have one-time training and never see [the trainer] again. But to see the continuity of the trainings and booster trainings, there is real opportunity for staff to attend these to feel more comfortable.

However, some interviewees also noted that the intensive nature of the MI Institute training, which was typically held off-site, was challenging to incorporate into their schedules, and some individuals reported discontinuing training due to these conflicts. In addition, for those who sought to hire external MI trainers, finding MI trainers that were culturally competent and able to provide both training and supervision was sometimes challenging. One MHP leader shared:

> The MI piece has been really complicated, the pay rate should be more of a supervisory level for the [MI trainer] someone that has experience coaching and working with others. I think that was very overwhelming for our [MI trainer], she had MI experience, but we didn't realize how hard it was to actually train and supervise MI, so that set us back and finding someone with those skills was really hard. I think that was stressful for [the CBO] and ourselves because we weren't coming through in that way.

Coaching and Supervision

As with initial training in C2C skills, CBOs and MHPs developed site-specific plans for implementing follow-up support (e.g., coaching sessions intended to reinforce skills for individuals that had previously completed training in the C2C skills) and supervision for CBO staff members that were trained in C2C. Coaching and supervision plans varied considerably based on CBO staff needs, CBO and MHP staff availability, MHP knowledge and capacity to implement supervisory systems for CBO staff, and preexisting supervisory systems within the CBO.

Nearly all sites incorporated ad hoc consultation in difficult or challenging cases, in which MHP staff were available by phone or in person to assist CBO staff with questions and concerns related to using the C2C skills with clients. Further, several sites also incorporated in-person shadowing and/or walk-in hours on-site for unscheduled coaching and supervisory sessions. Many sites also held more formal monthly or quarterly "booster trainings" for staff to provide a more structured environment in which staff members could ask questions and hone their skills.

Some sites opted to incorporate supervision and coaching for the C2C skills into preexisting supervisory activities for staff members (e.g., meetings in which staff supervisees meet with supervisors to discuss performance on a range of job activities in addition to delivery of C2C skills). In contrast, other CBOs explicitly separated supervision and coaching for C2C from supervision on other job activities.

Nearly all sites incorporated some form of group supervision for staff members who delivered C2C skills to clients. Although formats varied by site, group supervision took the form of supervisor-facilitated group meetings in which staff were encouraged to share experiences delivering C2C mental health supports to clients, provide supportive feedback, and discuss challenges and lessons-learned.

CBOs received extensive technical assistance surrounding development of coaching and supervision systems. Through program monitoring and technical assistance provided in year 1, the C2C Collaborative determined that many sites were experiencing challenges with establishing robust coaching and supervision structures for CBO staff members who delivered C2C mental health supports. In most instances, such challenges were attributable to uncertainty on the part of CBOs/MHPs regarding expectations for coaching and supervision, such as the frequency of coaching and supervision and methods for assessing and ensuring fidelity to best practices.

In response to these challenges, the C2C collaborative issued specific clarifying guidance in year 2 (May 2017), which required that staff members who deliver C2C receive C2C-specific supervision at least once per quarter (i.e., once every three months). The guidance also specified that targeted CBO staff and supervisors ($n = 409$) receive continuous coaching and supervision on a quarterly basis; this continuous coaching and supervision includes receiving reflective supervision twice per quarter, feedback based on direct practice observation once per quarter, and a coaching session related to a specific C2C skill once per quarter. Most CBOs were still in the process of refining and implementing revised supervision and coaching activities for C2C staff during year 2, especially at the time of evaluation interviews. However, the number of CBO staff and supervisors receiving continuous coaching and supervision increased over year 2— from 192 (47 percent of target) in the first quarter to 412 (101 percent of target) in the last quarter.

Figure 3.7 shows the number of coaching hours provided to CBO staff over time, based on CBO quarterly report data. MHPs and CBOs spent a total of 2,110 hours between March 2016 and March 2018 providing coaching in the core C2C skills. Following the clarification in coaching and supervision requirements in May 2017, coaching increased dramatically, with 78 percent of total hours occurring in year 2. As shown in Figure 3.7, MHPs delivered a majority (73 percent) of coaching hours in year 1 of the implementation process (CBO staff delivered 27 percent of total hours). Over time, CBOs and MHPs sought to expand the coaching capacity of on-site CBO management/supervisory staff members to increase in-house support for CBO direct service staff. Consistent with this, CBO staff members began to provide more coaching toward the end of year 2, with MHPs providing 56 percent and CBOs providing 44 percent of hours of total coaching hours. Such efforts may have been driven in part by a perceived need for additional on-site coaching for CBO staff who delivered C2C skills in year 1 (see *Staff Perceptions of Coaching and Supervision* below).

Figure 3.7. Number of Coaching Hours Provided by MHP and CBO, by Core C2C Skill

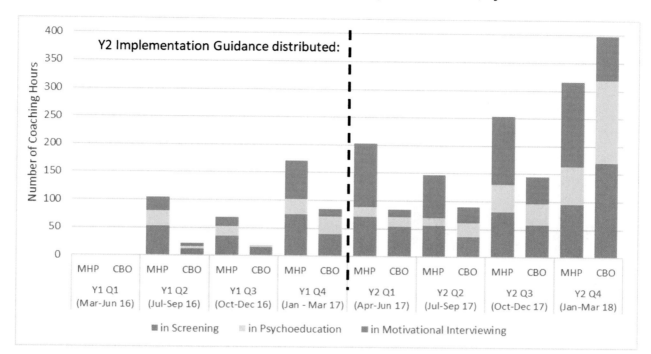

SOURCE: Data from quarterly CBO reports provided to RAND staff, 2016–2018.

Figure 3.8 shows survey data on staff member reports of supervision and coaching sources as of summer 2017. Approximately two-thirds of respondents indicated that they had received either group or one-on-one supervision or coaching from someone (i.e., a CBO or MHP staff member) with a formal education in a mental health–related field (e.g., a psychologist or licensed clinical social worker), whereas over 23 percent endorsed receiving supervision or coaching from a non–mental health specialist. Approximately 42 percent endorsed having some other type of supervision or coaching (e.g., peer supervision, CBO team meetings during which C2C skills were discussed).

Figure 3.8. Percentage of CBO Staff Who Received Coaching and Supervision in C2C Skills from Mental Health Professionals, Non–Mental Health Professionals, and Peers or Others

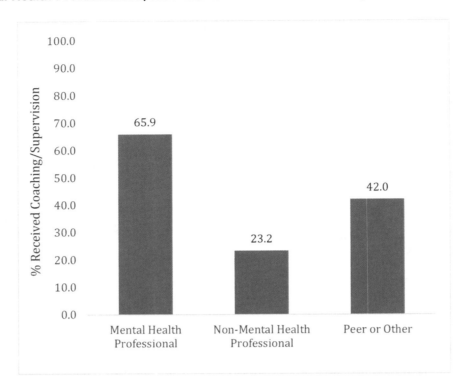

SOURCE: Data provided through annual survey of CBO staff, 2017.

In the early stages of C2C implementation (i.e., through the middle of year 2), there was considerable variability in the frequency of supervision and coaching for C2C staff. As shown in Figure 3.9, nearly half (46 percent) of staff survey respondents reported that they had received coaching or supervision once or twice since completing initial trainings, one-third (31 percent) reported receiving coaching or supervision between three and ten times, and 17 percent reported that they had never received coaching or supervision. Very few respondents (6 percent) reported receiving coaching or supervision more than ten times. Frequency of coaching and supervision varied based upon the type of training received. For example, among individuals who only received training in MHFA and answered the question about supervision frequency ($n = 20$), 30 percent reported that they had never received coaching and supervision, and 70 percent said they had received supervision at least once. In contrast, among individuals who received training in all four skills and answered the supervision frequency question ($n = 47$), 9 percent reported never receiving coaching or supervision, and 91 percent said they received it at least once. Of note, these data should be interpreted with caution, as data collection occurred shortly after initial trainings in some cases and at a time when many organizations were in the process of developing or strengthening implementation of coaching or supervision programs. Moreover, survey data were collected shortly after distribution of clarifying guidance in May 2017 surrounding coaching and supervision requirements. The second wave of survey data collection is currently

50

under way, and updated information on coaching and supervision—as well as progress toward quarterly continuous coaching and supervision targets set after revised guidance was issued—will be presented in the forthcoming final evaluation report.

Figure 3.9. Frequency of Coaching or Supervision Sessions Reported by Staff

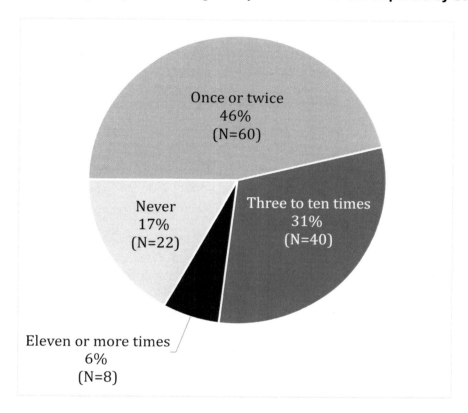

SOURCE: Data provided through annual survey of CBO staff, 2017.

Staff Perceptions of Coaching and Supervision

As with initial trainings, many staff reported favorable views of coaching and supervision as of summer 2017. However, most CBO staff members expressed a desire for more coaching and supervisory support. About half (47 percent) of survey respondents agreed or strongly agreed with the statement "I am satisfied with the supervision I have received in C2C mental health modalities," and two-thirds of respondents (66 percent) agreed with the statement "I could use additional training, coaching, and/or supervision in C2C mental health modalities."

Similarly, desire for more coaching and supervision—as well as booster training—was a common theme in staff key informant interviews conducted in summer 2017, although some individuals acknowledged scheduling time for additional support as a potential barrier. For example, one staff member stated:

> I think if there was more contact and more practice, I would feel better about it but—once again, it's hard because we're all so busy all of the time and, of

course, it would be beneficial to have more trainings, more booster sessions, more refreshers, but it's just hard sometimes.

CBO staff and leaders also shared additional barriers to coaching and supervision. For example, logistical barriers such as scheduling conflicts and MHP's limited availability made coaching and supervision challenging. In response, some MHP trainers offered flexible coaching and supervision opportunities. An MHP trainer shared:

> We [CBO staff and trainer] are thinking at least once a month for us to have [coaching and supervision] because of just continuity of them being able to practice. Also, I do have open office hours here, so staff are aware that they can make an appointment with me and we can work on whatever it is that they feel like they want to work on. They know that the support is there, and they know when they can access it and they can reach me.

As noted above with respect to C2C trainings, efforts to incorporate staff experiences into ongoing coaching and supervision activities (e.g., through role play exercises) were seen as particularly helpful for staff. In addition, coaching and supervision sessions that included reflective supervision were well received by CBO staff. When asked about what aspects of supervision were most helpful, one CBO staff said:

> The reflection—our supervisor asks us how we reacted and managed through different conversations or situations that we experience with clients.

Staff Readiness to Deliver C2C

CBO and MHP leadership put forth considerable effort to ensure that staff felt comfortable and confident in their use of C2C skills with clients prior to delivering them. Messaging C2C to staff and ensuring strong staff buy-in were viewed as important components for ensuring staff readiness to use C2C skills with clients. For example, some CBO leaders presented C2C as a way to equip staff with skills and tools to better serve the clients. As described by one CBO lead:

> I think it's been about empowering staff because they [staff] are really the ones who are meeting and speaking to participants every single day. So, providing them with the proper tools to have conversations with participations, I think that has been a key component to engage participants in services.

CBO and MHP leaders also reported that staff buy-in has improved since C2C was first introduced in most sites. This was largely viewed as a product of efforts to tailor training and support to meet staff needs, and to incorporate their feedback. One MHP leader discussed the improvement in staff buy-in:

> In year 1, staff wasn't sure what the point was or how the instruments were going to work. But I think this year, they [staff] are very engaged, the administration here has been very supportive, very engaged, so in seeing the importance of this, that has been very nice.

The training and support provided to staff members helped them to increase buy-in and confidence to deliver C2C to clients. One CBO leader shared:

I think the training aspect of it there's definitely more buy-in; they [staff] are responding, they're using it when they come talk to me individually. If they had a certain experience with a client, they know that the support is there.

As shown in Figure 3.10, as of summer 2017, about half of staff members endorsed feeling confident in using the C2C skills in which they had been trained with their clients. This suggests that while many staff may have felt ready to use their new C2C skills, a substantial proportion did not yet feel confident. Further, confidence ratings varied across C2C support types; respondents tended to be somewhat less confident in their ability to deliver psychoeducation compared with the other four supports. This may be attributable in part to changes in guidance for psychoeducation that were enacted in year 2, when additional requirements to use evidence-based, structured psychoeducation programs were put forth. At the time of the survey, most sites were in the process of revising their approach to conform to this guidance. In addition, because the survey was conducted early in the implementation process, respondents may have had limited experience in utilizing C2C skills with clients.

Figure 3.10. Percentage of Staff Endorsing Confidence in Using C2C Skills with Clients

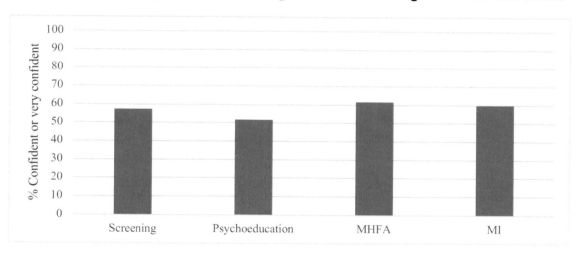

SOURCE: Data provided through annual survey of CBO staff, 2017.

Most staff members who completed the annual survey also reported high awareness of and access to resources to help clients with mental health concerns (see Figure 3.11). For example, 81 percent of respondents agreed or strongly agreed with the statement "I can identify the places or people where I should refer clients experiencing behavioral health difficulties." In addition, nearly three-quarters of respondents (74 percent) agreed that they were equipped with adequate resources at their organizations to facilitate referrals for clients with behavioral health difficulties. A majority of staff members (83 percent) also endorsed that they felt encouraged by their organization to talk to clients about behavioral health difficulties.

Figure 3.11. Staff Preparedness to Help Clients with Behavioral Health Issues and Access to Organizational Supports

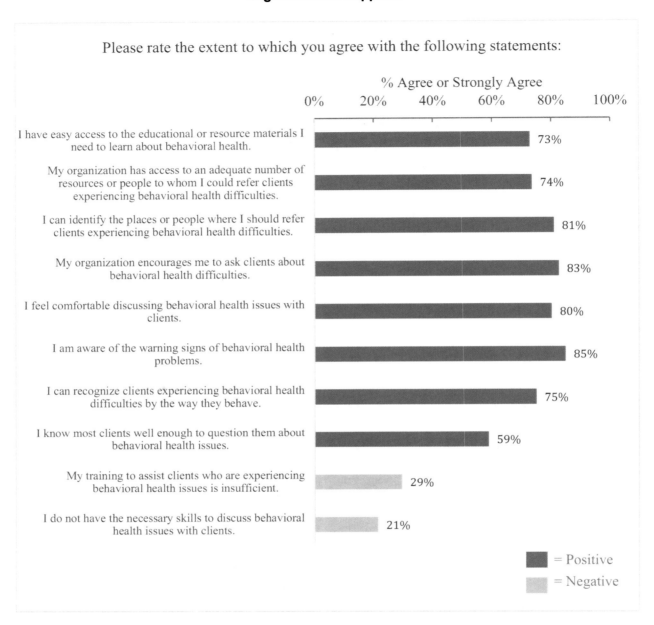

SOURCE: Data provided through annual survey of CBO staff, 2017.

Although many staff members expressed confidence in using the C2C skills with clients, some interviewees expressed initial discomfort talking to clients about mental health issues and were less confident than their peers in their ability to deliver the C2C skills. One CBO staff member said:

> You know—it is somewhat intimidating. . . . My comfort level is somewhat
> tested when someone then opens up and says all what they're feeling. I'll look

through the notes and be like *"we didn't cover this* [in training]." . . . I feel like I'm limited without a background in mental health.

However, staff—particularly those with no prior experience in a mental health–related field—expressed that opportunities to practice using the C2C skills with clients, along with ongoing coaching and supervision, were helpful in improving staff members' confidence to discuss mental health issues and use the C2C skills with clients. For example, a CBO staff member said:

> [The MHP liaison] helped me get the conversation flowing because I didn't know what I was doing. It was helpful to learn how to initiate that conversation. So honestly, it taught me how to open up the conversation. And she sat me down with multiple clients, trying to teach me how to do [psychoeducation], and she taught me the process. So now I'm more confident in talking to them.

C2C Service Delivery

Client Receipt of C2C Services

Between March 2016 and March 2018 (year 1 and year 2), a total of 16,701 unique clients across 15 CBOs received C2C mental health services, according to CBO quarterly report data. Clients receiving C2C mental health services are defined as those who got screening, psychoeducation, referral to an MHP or other mental health provider, and/or engaged with a CBO staff person trained to deliver one or more C2C skill. MI and MHFA were determined to be too difficult to quantify for the purposes of the CBO quarterly reports. Figure 3.12 shows the cumulative number of clients served through C2C based on quarterly report data submitted by CBOs over the course of implementation. Across all CBOs during the first two years of implementation, an average of 3,443 clients per quarter received a C2C mental health service (note that individual clients may have received services in more than one quarter). At the end of year 1, CBOs had reached 59 percent of their target (8,662) for new C2C clients. However, in year 2, CBOs reached 177 percent of their target (8,454). Cumulatively, CBOs have reached 98 percent of their total (years 1 and 2) target of 17,116 new clients.

Figure 3.12. Cumulative Number of C2C Program Clients, C2C Years 1 and 2

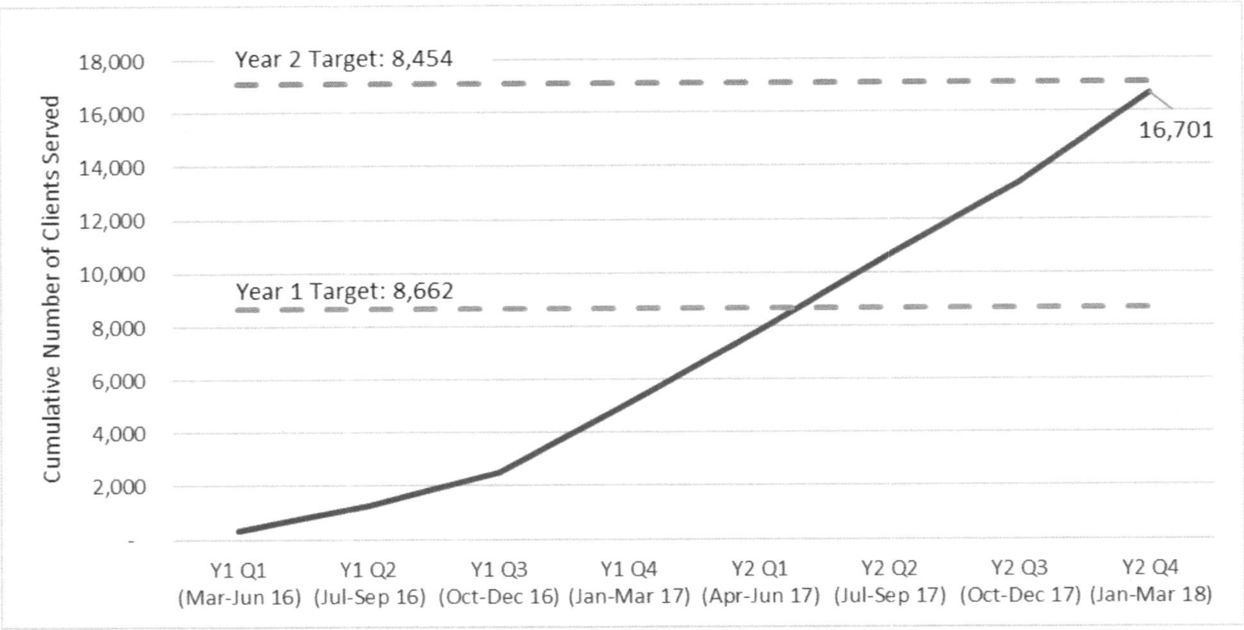

SOURCE: Data from quarterly CBO reports provided to RAND staff, 2016–2018.

Table 3.1 shows a breakdown of demographic information for all clients who received any C2C supports. These data should be interpreted with caution, as there are high rates of unreported and missing data for each category, particularly for year 1 data (when many organizations were in the process of updating their data systems to accommodate collection and reporting of these and other metrics).

Table 3.1. Demographic Characteristics of C2C Clients

	N	%
Gender		
Male (incl. trans)	6,757	40.5
Female (incl. trans)	6,595	39.5
Other	171	1.0
Unreported/missing	3,178	19.0
Age		
16–17	1,447	8.7
18–24	5,737	34.4
25–44	4,666	27.9
45–64	1,434	8.6
65+	58	0.3
Unreported/missing	3,359	20.1
Ethnicity		
Hispanic	4,979	29.8
Non-Hispanic	7,828	46.9
Unreported/missing	3,894	23.3
Race		
Black	6,886	41.2
White	714	4.3
Asian/Pacific Islander	306	1.8
Other	4,708	28.2
Unreported/missing	4,087	24.5
Education Status		
Less than high school	5,817	34.8
High school degree	4,006	24.0
Some college/vocational (no degree completed)	1,181	7.1
College/vocational degree or higher	904	5.4
Unreported/missing	4,793	28.7
Employment Status		
Full-time	1,351	8.1
Part-time	1,251	7.5
Not employed	7,812	46.8
Unreported/missing	6,287	37.6

SOURCE: Data from quarterly CBO reports provided to RAND staff, 2016–2018.

Figure 3.13 shows the number of C2C clients receiving supports over the first two years. Early in the implementation process, nearly all organizations prioritized implementation of MHFA and screening for CBO clients over delivery of other types of support. However, in year 2, more clients received at least one of the other supports (i.e., psychoeducation, MI). An average of 46 percent of all CBO clients met with a C2C-trained CBO or MHP staff person (i.e., received screening, receiving psychoeducation, had an encounter with a staff member trained in MHFA or MI). However, this overall average masks the substantial increase in the percentage of CBO clients receiving C2C supports over time, from an average of 22 percent in year 1 to 70 percent in year 2.

Figure 3.13. Number of Clients Who Received C2C Skills Each Quarter

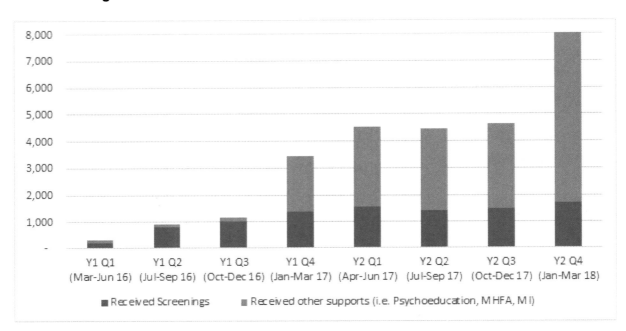

SOURCE: Data from quarterly CBO reports provided to RAND staff, 2016–2018.

Over the first two years of C2C implementation, 9,618 clients received behavioral health screening. While it did not appear that CBOs applied systematic re-screening of clients at this stage of implementation, clients may have been screened in multiple quarters. On average (i.e., mean of percentages across all quarters), half (50 percent) of C2C clients were screened each quarter. As shown in Figure 3.14, number of screenings increased steadily during implementation scale-up in year 1 before stabilizing in year 2. Moreover, the number of clients reached by other C2C skills (psychoeducation, MHFA, MI) increased considerably toward the end of year 2, consistent with sites' emphasis on training and implementing supports such as MI and psychoeducation during that year.

Figure 3.14. Number of Clients Screened for Behavioral Health Symptoms

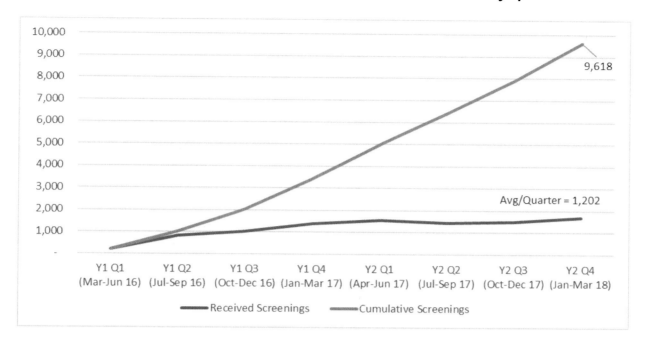

Screening content (i.e., type of behavioral health issue) and specific instruments varied across organizations, based on perceived needs of CBOs' target client populations. Moreover, delivery of a single screening "battery" could include multiple instruments. Figure 3.15 shows the number of clients who were screened. Among clients who received behavioral health screening (9,618 clients; a total of 17,122 screening surveys), 2,833 clients (30 percent) screened positive in one or more screening surveys. This positive screening rate is consistent with findings from epidemiological studies of similar populations. For example, the prevalence of mood disorders and anxiety among lower-income populations were found to be 15 percent and 25 percent, respectively (Muntaner et al., 1998). As shown in the figure, depression was the most common behavioral health issue for which CBOs screened clients, followed by substance abuse, anxiety, and PTSD. Although not required by the C2C model, seven CBOs chose to implement screens for PTSD. Among clients screened, PTSD was the most common behavioral health issue for which clients screened positive, with nearly 36 percent of those screened having possibly significant PTSD symptoms. In addition, about one-fourth (23 percent) of clients screened for anxiety had positive results. Approximately one-fifth of clients (20 percent) screened positive for potentially serious depressive symptoms that could benefit from treatment, and one-tenth of clients screened positive for substance use disorder (11 percent).

Figure 3.15. Total Number of Behavioral Health Screenings, by Symptom Category

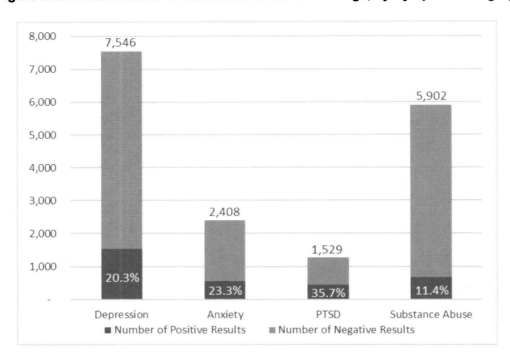

SOURCE: Data from quarterly CBO reports provided to RAND staff, 2016–2018.

A total of 2,254 clients accepted a referral to behavioral health providers through the C2C program; 89 percent of referrals were to the MHP, and 11 percent of referrals were to external providers. Almost 60 percent (n = 1,333) of clients referred kept an appointment. Clients may have received external (i.e., non-MHP) referrals for a number of reasons, including, but not limited to, client preference or treatment needs, location/travel consideration, insurance and/or payment considerations, and scheduling considerations. Of note, while positive screening results were a primary mechanism used to prompt referrals, clients did not need to screen positive—nor complete a screening— to receive a referral. For example, in year 2, 1,037 clients (51 percent of positive screens) were referred to the MHP or an external provider after screening positive, and an additional 501 clients were referred based on other prompts (e.g., client request, staff identification of a client behavioral health concern). In addition, 615 clients (30 percent of positive screens) declined a referral after screening positive, and 166 clients declined referrals provided based on other prompts. Clients may have declined referrals for a variety of reasons that may not necessarily indicate unmet treatment need (e.g., client is already in treatment, client is not interested in treatment at the time, client is able to address needs through working with CBO staff).

Figure 3.16 shows the cumulative number of clients referred to treatment over time. Similar to screenings, cumulative client referrals have increased in a relatively linear fashion over the course of C2C implementation to date. These numbers should be interpreted with caution, however, as data likely do not reflect the full scope of individuals who were *offered* a referral (i.e., all formal or informal referral attempts made by CBO staff, which may not have been documented systematically) but rather only reflect formal accepted referrals documented by staff. In addition, some clients who were referred to treatment and missed an initial appointment may have attended an appointment at a later date and/or declined to share attendance information with the CBO.

Figure 3.16. Cumulative Number of Clients Referred to Mental Health Treatment

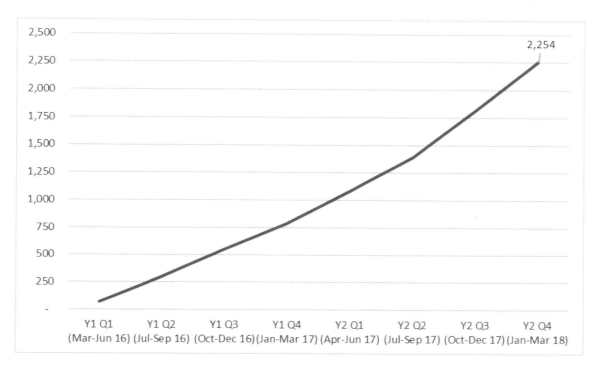

SOURCE: Data from quarterly CBO reports provided to RAND staff, 2016–2018.

Figure 3.17 shows the total number of individuals who were referred to treatment each quarter, as well as the number of those clients who were confirmed to have attended at least one appointment with a behavioral health provider. On average, across all quarters, approximately 59 percent of clients referred to treatment attended at least one appointment with a provider. This completion rate varied across CBOs, ranging from 14 percent to 100 percent (median = 58 percent). Six CBOs met the target of 70 percent referral completion rate that was set by the C2C Collaborative. Follow-up procedures with CBO clients (i.e., individuals who declined initial referral may or may not be offered a second referral) and use of strategies to improve engagement (e.g., use of and capacity to conduct warm handoffs) varied considerably across CBOs. Sites have received ongoing technical assistance throughout the implementation process to augment referral practices and to help navigate challenges with completing client referrals. One thing that is unclear is how many sessions individuals attended following an initial appointment. More detailed information on screening, referrals, and treatment utilization will be

61

collected as part of the impact evaluation, and these results will be presented in the forthcoming full evaluation report in 2020.

Figure 3.17. Number of Clients Who Completed Referrals, by Quarter

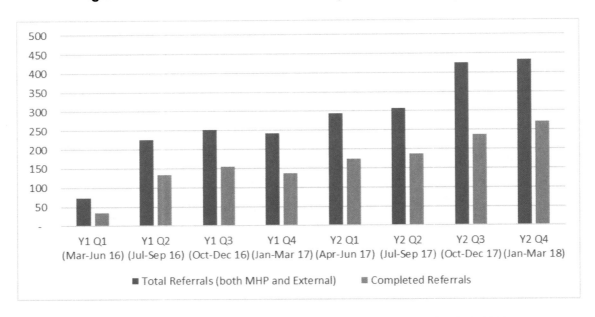

SOURCE: Data from quarterly CBO reports provided to RAND staff, 2016–2018.

Key informant interviews highlighted a range of potential barriers with getting clients to accept referrals, but also identified a number of strategies to overcome these challenges and facilitate client referrals. For example, MHP leaders highlighted organizational policies and procedures with respect to visit scheduling and attendance (e.g., a "three strikes" rule whereby clients who are scheduled and fail to attend three appointments are moved to the bottom of the appointment wait list) as potential barriers to providing services to referred clients. In response to these challenges, many MHPs tried to be flexible and to meet the needs of clients and modify organizational factors to improve access to CBO clients. In some cases, MHP efforts to accommodate CBO clients for C2C involved changes to standard practices or procedures. As discussed by one MHP:

> We try to be flexible with appointment times when people are available. We have the social workers from [the CBO] accompany [clients] to our clinic for their intake appointment, and we reschedule appointments that we would not normally reschedule.

Similarly, another MHP leader discussed efforts to facilitate warm hand-offs and modify intake procedures to accommodate CBO client referrals in more detail:

> We had to develop protocol for doing that. I do intakes here [at CBO] instead of referring the person to [the MHP] and having it happen there, so when the client gets to [the MHP], the intake and other necessary paperwork is done, and they

62

can meet with their therapist . . . . So, we've had a streamlining of the referral process and that's been a more effective way of doing it . . . [also] when they're backed up at [the MHP], we close intakes for a minute—but they're never closed to [CBO] clients. They're always open to them and prioritized.

Client-related barriers, especially perceived stigma associated with mental health conditions, limited resources (e.g., lack of insurance, lack of transportation), and privacy concerns, were viewed as having a negative effect on referral completion. Many CBO leaders and staff stated that several of their clients and their communities view mental health treatment in a negative light and are not comfortable with seeking mental health treatment or discussing mental health issues. One CBO leader shared:

> Trying to push clients to come and see [social worker] in the referral process— that's the other layer, which is the stigma within our communities. . . . I think that's the biggest barrier—for folks to come and actually see a social worker. People are just not really used to mental health services.

Clients' limited ability to access treatment, including lack of transportation, lack of health insurance, financial constraints, and lack of child care for parents, were the most commonly cited client resource-related barriers to referral acceptance. One MHP leader shared:

> There are a lot of barriers like the metro card and getting there. I'm thinking of a [client] that was homeless and was kind of couch surfing [with] two kids—one in school and one in daycare, no family support, and it's like "What do I do with my kids? How do I get out there? I'm worried about my next meal and where I'm going to sleep." So, there are a lot of barriers that come up, but I think we've done a pretty good job of trying to resolve them or neutralize them.

Many CBOs and MHPs actively worked together to address these types of challenges to improve clients' ability to access mental health resources. For example, CBOs and MHPs provided transit cards, expanded MHP office hours, and gave appointment priorities to C2C clients at MHP clinics (i.e., CBO clients were given first available appointments). Some CBO interviewees discussed the possibility of adding or expanding MHP staff onsite to facilitate clients' access to services: "We are working on having a satellite site [at the CBO] for counseling so that the counselors are available onsite. . . . We figured maybe if we bring it to where the clients are, they are more likely to use it."

Clients' concerns about confidentiality and mistrust toward mental health professionals were also barriers to C2C implementation. Several clients shared that they have trouble trusting mental health service providers due to negative past experiences. In response to a question about previous experience with mental health services, one client said:

> I was in high school, so I was kind of forced to check it out. Terrible experience—there was this one person that said they kept things confidential. I trusted and told her everything that was happening, and she told someone else about what I shared.

Positive relationships between CBO staff members and clients helped ease these concerns for some clients. Clients' trust in CBO staff was described as critical for implementing C2C skills.

For example, a client said, "I talk to people here because I trust them, and I don't trust people very much." Another client shared:

> They work here, but they make you feel like it's family—and if you're not comfortable here they will make you get comfortable here. They just opened me up to talk more, because when I first got here I didn't really want to talk, and I was like "I don't know all these people" but they treat you like family, so they really open you up.

In an effort to reduce barriers to engaging in behavioral health treatment, CBO and MHP staff members actively communicated with clients about their concerns and educated clients about behavioral health treatment. As noted by one MHP staff member:

> I present the idea of seeking care and the first thing I usually hear is "I'm not seeing a psychiatrist!". . . Psycho-education is important. In [psychoeducation training workshops] we have a handout about the therapy experience, and it does distinguish the different types of mental health providers. So just giving these people this information is really empowering, so they can decide the type of provider they want to see.

Additionally, some organizations broke down barriers to client referrals through efforts to familiarize clients with MHP (and non-MHP clinic) settings:

> We have identified resources and partners around the community, so we are starting to take trips out to these other agencies so that clients can see what those places look like and they are not as suspicious to follow a referral.

Staff Time Spent Delivering C2C

After receiving training in C2C mental health practices, CBO staff members reported using these new skills regularly during their interactions with clients. Figure 3.18 shows staff respondents' ($n = 140$) self-reported proportion of clients with whom they used any C2C support. A majority of respondents (51 percent) reported using at least one C2C support with many, almost all, or all of the clients they served.

Figure 3.18. Proportion of Clients to Whom Staff Members Have Delivered Any C2C Skill

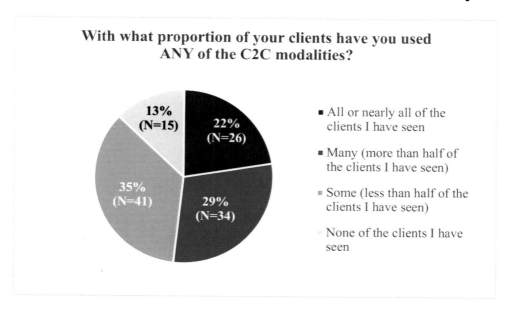

With what proportion of your clients have you used
ANY of the C2C modalities?

- 13% (N=15)
- 22% (N=26)
- 35% (N=41)
- 29% (N=34)

- All or nearly all of the clients I have seen
- Many (more than half of the clients I have seen)
- Some (less than half of the clients I have seen)
- None of the clients I have seen

SOURCE: Data provided through annual survey of CBO staff, 2017.

According to staff survey data, the frequency with which staff used the different core C2C mental health supports with clients varied. Among individuals trained in screening, over half (61 percent) reported either never (24 percent) or rarely (37 percent) delivering that support. Similarly, among individuals trained in MHFA, most (69 percent) reported never, rarely, or sometimes using it with clients. In contrast, for those trained in psychoeducation, only 13 percent reported never delivering the support to clients, and nearly half (43 percent) reported using psychoeducation regularly to frequently with clients. Finally, nearly two-thirds of staff (63 percent) trained in MI reported delivering the support regularly, often, or frequently. Such variability aligns with differences in implementation plans across organizations but, as noted above, at the time of the survey, CBOs also varied considerably with respect to when each C2C support had been initiated. Additionally, some organizations provided training to staff members who had limited direct contact with clients (e.g., leadership, management) and/or were not expected to provide all types of mental health supports to clients on a regular basis. For example, some staff may have participated in trainings for screening for informational purposes (e.g., to know how to interpret screening data) or to serve as backup for one or two staff members who were tasked with regularly administering screenings as part of intake procedures.

CBO staff reported devoting a considerable amount of time each week to using C2C mental health skills with clients. Figure 3.19 shows the amount of time that staff members spent delivering C2C mental health skills and referring clients to behavioral health services (i.e., to an MHP, to an external provider) in a typical work week. Consistent with training and implementation models, direct service staff and client-facing staff reported spending the most time engaging in C2C-related activities with clients—more than eight hours per week on average. Of note, this does not necessarily reflect *additional* time spent with clients on top of typical job responsibilities; rather, C2C-related activities may have been integrated into regular work activities (e.g., intake procedures, workshops, client meetings).

Figure 3.19. Hours Per Week Spent Delivering C2C and Referring Clients to MHPs

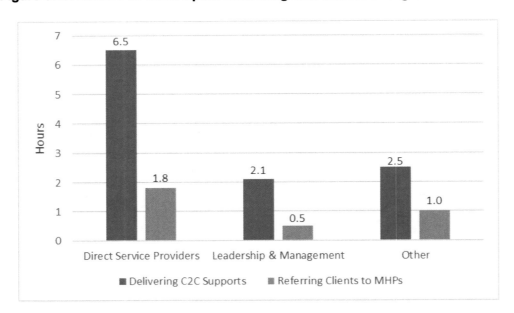

In addition, staff members reported on specific types of helping behaviors that they used while interacting with clients who had mental health and substance use issues. Figure 3.20 shows the proportion of survey respondents who reported that they always or almost always engaged in a number of different behaviors when they suspected or knew that a client was experiencing mental health problems. Nearly all staff members (91 percent) reported that they would always or almost always spend time listening to a client in such instances. However, only about two-thirds of staff (61 percent) reported that they would *ask* the client about mental health issues, suggesting that—at the time of the survey in early year 2—a sizable minority of staff members may still have been reluctant to engage clients in conversations about mental health. Engagement in other helping behaviors varied. For example, over three-quarters of staff (77 percent) reported that, when they suspect a client is experiencing a mental health issue, they always or almost always provide clients with information about behavioral health and/or how to get help. Over half of staff members (54 percent) also reported that they always or almost always assist clients with behavioral health difficulties by escorting the client to a counselor or some other mental health resource. Such variability may also correspond to situational differences (e.g., whether this is a crisis situation, client presentation and preferences). The forthcoming final report will examine changes in such self-reported behaviors over the course of the implementation process.

Figure 3.20. Staff Use of Specific Helping Behaviors with Clients

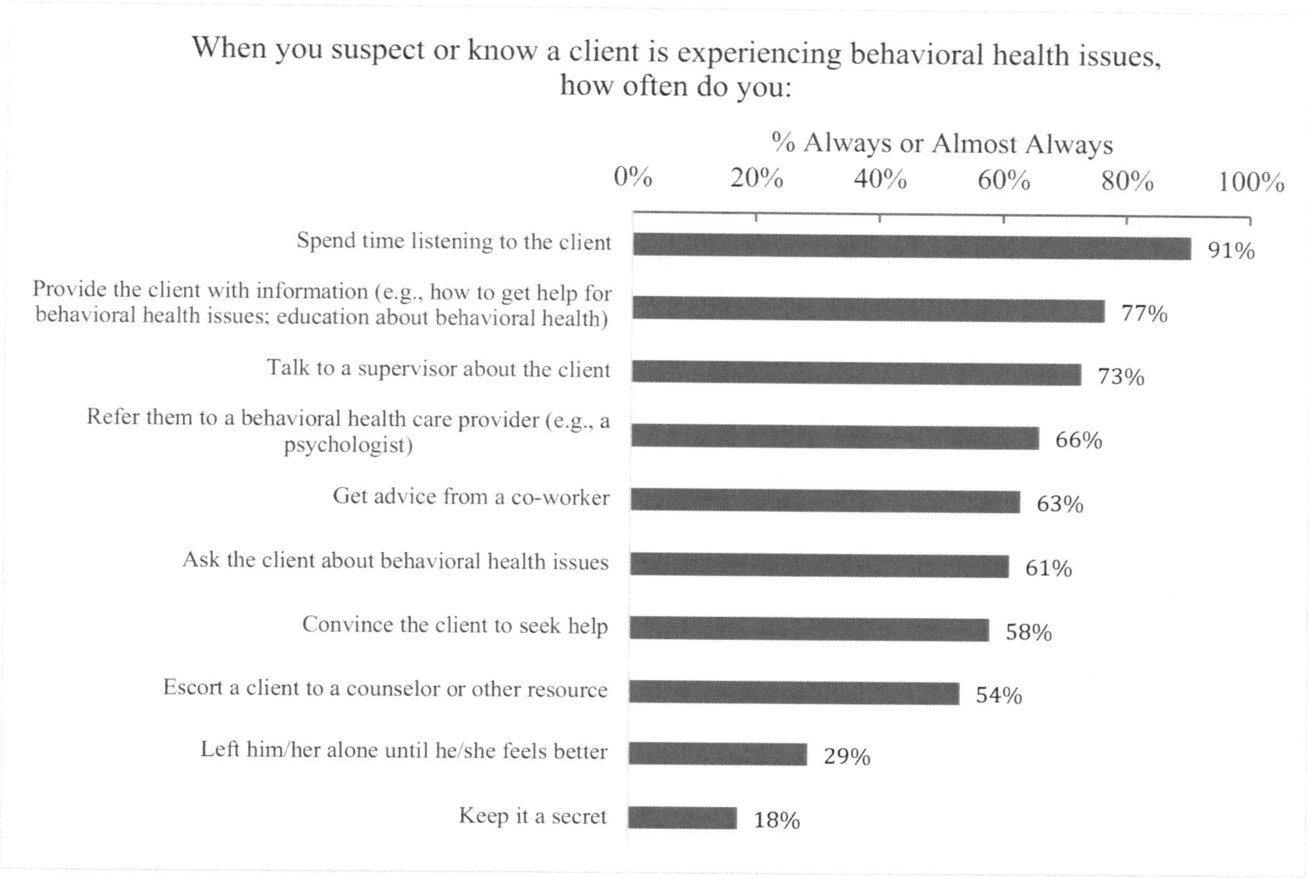

When you suspect or know a client is experiencing behavioral health issues, how often do you:

% Always or Almost Always

Behavior	%
Spend time listening to the client	91%
Provide the client with information (e.g., how to get help for behavioral health issues; education about behavioral health)	77%
Talk to a supervisor about the client	73%
Refer them to a behavioral health care provider (e.g., a psychologist)	66%
Get advice from a co-worker	63%
Ask the client about behavioral health issues	61%
Convince the client to seek help	58%
Escort a client to a counselor or other resource	54%
Left him/her alone until he/she feels better	29%
Keep it a secret	18%

SOURCE: Data provided through annual survey of CBO staff, 2017.

Perceived Impact of C2C

Although the C2C program was still in the early stages of implementation during the first round of key informant interviews, many interviewees highlighted some early positive impacts of C2C on CBOs, MHPs, and clients. CBO leaders and staff members discussed improvements in their approach to addressing clients' mental health issues. Some interviewees credited C2C for cultural shifts in how their organization began to recognize the importance of mental health. One CBO leader said:

> We are more comprehensive in our service delivery so we're not just approaching a participant or client and evaluating [progress in the CBO program]. We're also going to ask about other aspects of their lives and have a place to refer them if it seems like they would benefit from seeing [social worker] or having counseling.

Moreover, many interviewees shared that C2C has given them a common language to discuss mental health issues and taught them new skills to address clients' mental health concerns. For example, a CBO leader said, "[C2C] is helping develop common language around mental health within our community, conversation around mental health has broadened, it can be more of a universal conversation among the staff."

CBO staff members also reported that C2C has provided them with a deeper understanding of the clients they serve and, in turn, changed the way they approach and interact with clients. For example:

> It's been, for me, like a light. Like turning on a light in a dark room. It opened my eyes and allowed me to better understand the individuals I work with and understand when they really need assistance and what kind they might need. And not just for our clients we work with, but for myself. It allows me—when I'm frustrated dealing with a person—to evaluate how I handle myself and know if it's time to remove myself. Or it allows me to say, "you need to move from point a to b" and to say it without making the individual feel like I'm judging them.

Some CBO leaders and staff members reported that both participation in C2C trainings and delivery of C2C skills to clients was beneficial to their own mental health and helped them with stress management. One CBO leader recalled a staff member saying, "you have no idea how much C2C and the trainings have helped me with my personal life." Another CBO staff member shared a personal experience:

> On a personal note, again, doing this job I'm very happy to have mental health within the programs and people to remind me to think about how *I'm feeling* . . . my job can be very stressful, so I'm very happy to have strategies and be reminded of other strategies and techniques. It feels nice to know that mental wellness is a very strong component in our program.

Some CBO leaders and staff also said that C2C has led to collaboration among participating CBOs and has facilitated sharing of resources, best practices, and curricula. One CBO leader discussed how the connection with other CBOs has benefited clients as well, saying:

> When you think about connecting and access for our clients across the spectrum to care, it's incredible what [C2C] is doing, because some of these organizations can support our [clients] in different ways and vice versa, so we're all wanting to visit each other's agencies and stay connected.

Some CBO leaders initiated formal gatherings to facilitate resources sharing among CBOs. One said, "I also kicked off a workforce group for C2C to learn how different providers who are working towards the same goal have achieved that. We kicked that off here and hopefully the community will keep it going." The large network of different CBOs within C2C and frequent contact between organizational leads allowed participating CBOs to learn from each other. "We would never have learned that without talking to other providers. We're able to *not* recreate the wheel and have shared learning."

Many interviewees reported that they thought their clients had benefited from C2C skills. C2C skills were described as improving clients' well-being, connection to additional services, and use of services. One CBO staff shared an experience with a client:

I had a client come to me and say, "there is seriously something wrong with me, I have no appetite," but then when we are doing the screening for depression and they saw some of their symptoms reflected, they were like, "ok, maybe I am experiencing depression, maybe I should go speak with someone."

CBO and MHP interviewees also discussed reducing stigma associated with mental health and normalizing the acceptance of mental health services as C2C benefits to clients. One MHP leader shared, "I think it is wonderful to see how many people come from the neighborhood that would never consider mental health services." Moreover, some CBO staff members said that C2C is helping some clients initiate conversations with CBO staff about needed services, and connect to treatment more quickly than they may have otherwise:

Sometimes it might take up to ten years for someone with mental illness to address that. We've found that we can cut some of that time for people we service. . . . Clients now are able to come to [staff] and say, "I think I'd like to see someone now." I'm not sure if that was available before C2C.

Clients also shared ways in which C2C has positively affected their lives. As stated by one client:

A friend told me about [CBO] and told me how great it was, and he found [it to be] a sanctuary almost. They met me down where I was . . . and helped me build my confidence . . . deal mentally with my emotions and what was going on at home and in my personal life. And then they referred me to counseling, so I feel like this is great—and the people are awesome!

In addition to improving their individual well-being, some clients discussed how C2C has helped with their relationships with family members:

This has singlehandedly made me a better parent . . . it's about my relationship with my child. I changed a lot, which in turn changed our relationship a lot . . . now she talks to me. I wasn't listening, so how I could I hear her?

Some clients also talked about ways in which C2C may be changing perspectives toward mental health and helping people to progress toward their goals. One said:

A lot of people think that mental help [mental health treatment] is for "crazies," but it's not. It's for people who need help to reach their full potential. . . . I would have never been able to move forward in life without my mental health.

Conclusions

Overall, preliminary findings from the C2C implementation evaluation indicate that, in years 1 and 2 of the program, CBOs and MHPs made considerable progress toward implementing multiple components of the C2C program. In the early stages of implementation, CBOs and MHPs strengthened relationships and learned about one another's organizations; implemented training and ongoing coaching/supervision for CBO staff in the four core C2C mental health skills; began delivering mental health supports to clients and referred many clients to more-intensive services at both C2C-affiliated MHPs and external providers; witnessed some preliminary changes in organizational culture toward mental health; and took steps to address barriers to connecting clients with mental health care. Data collection for the implementation evaluation is ongoing, and findings from later stages of the implementation process—and changes over time—will be detailed in the forthcoming final report in 2020.

4. Interim Impact Evaluation Progress and Baseline Descriptive Data

In this chapter, we describe early progress and provide some baseline descriptive data from the impact evaluation. It is important to note that data collection is ongoing and study enrollment is only about halfway complete at the time of this writing. Thus, the numbers presented here will change and should not be taken as final; the data presented in this chapter should be interpreted simply as a "snapshot" of the sample midway through data collection.

As noted earlier, 13 C2C CBOs and ten comparison group CBOs are participating in the impact evaluation (Table 4.1). CBOs were categorized by their primary offering or organizational type: workforce development, youth development, early childhood development, homeless shelters, domestic violence organizations, and agencies serving Hispanic/Latino adults. The number of CBOs in each category is detailed in Table 4.1. Many of the CBOs, both C2C and comparison, have multiple sites involved in the study. Across the 13 C2C CBOs, clients are being enrolled at 23 sites. At the ten comparison CBOs, data are being collected at 16 sites. As described in Chapters 1 and 2, the impact evaluation uses survey and demographic data on C2C participants and clients of comparison CBOs to gauge the effect of the C2C program on participant outcomes, both between groups and over time.

Table 4.1. CBO Information

Category	C2C CBOs	Comparison CBOs
Workforce development	5	3*
Youth development	3	3*
Early childhood development	2	1*
Homeless shelter	1	1
Domestic violence organizations	1	1
Agency serving Hispanic/Latino adults	1	1

* One comparison CBO recruits study participants from both a workforce development program and a youth development program; one comparison CBO recruits study participants from both a workforce development program and an early childhood development program.

Client Survey

As described in Chapter 2, to be eligible, participants must have screened positive on at least one of the five screeners. As of July 31, 2018, 1,234 C2C eligibility screenings have been completed, 65 percent of which were from the C2C group and 35 percent from the comparison group (Table 4.2).

Table 4.2. Status of Data Collection as of July 31, 2018

	Total	C2C	Comparison
Completed screenings	1,234	805	429
Eligible based on screenings	1,047 (85%)	693 (86%)	354 (83%)
Completed baseline surveys	901 (86%)	634 (91%)	267 (75%)

Recruitment for participants from the C2C CBOs started earlier than comparison CBOs, as the latter entered into agreements with us later in the course of the project. Overall, 85 percent of individuals screened were eligible for the study, meaning scores met the minimum threshold for at least one of the five measures on the eligibility screener (see Appendix A). As described in Chapter 2, a lower threshold on the study eligibility screening measures was used in comparison with thresholds used for clinical purposes because this study is focused on individuals with a range of symptom severity and is not limited to those with a possible clinical diagnosis. Individuals who screened as eligible were offered the opportunity to participate in the study. Baseline surveys were completed for 86 percent of eligible screens overall, above the target of 80 percent of eligibility screens; therefore, study enrollment also exceeded its target. The baseline completion rate was somewhat higher at C2C CBOs (91 percent) than comparison group CBOs (75 percent).

Demographic Data

Table 4.3 provides a summary of baseline demographics for the sample of C2C study participants (totals may add up to more than 100 percent due to rounding.) We chose not to present comparison group data in this interim report in order to prevent premature interpretation of any C2C-comparison group differences, given that study enrollment is ongoing through March 2019. In the C2C group, about one-half identify as female; 49 percent as male; and 2 percent as transgender, genderqueer, or some other gender identity. About 40 percent of the C2C study participants were 18 to 24 at the time of the baseline survey, 15 percent were 25 to 30 years of age, and 18 percent were 31 to 40 years of age; almost one-quarter (23 percent) of the C2C study participants were over 40 at the time of the baseline survey. A small percentage of C2C study participants (4 percent) were less than 18 years of age at baseline. A substantial minority (39 percent) of the C2C study participants identified as Hispanic/Latino. The majority of study participants (56 percent) identified as Black/African American, with smaller percentages identifying as White/Caucasian (7 percent), American Indian or Alaskan Native (2 percent), or Asian or Pacific Islander (1 percent). Eighteen percent identified as "other race"; another 18 percent did not provide a response. The education level of C2C participants at baseline ranged from less than high school (30 percent) to completed graduate or professional school (2 percent). Just over one-third (34 percent) had completed high school with a diploma or General Equivalency Development (GED) diploma at the time of the baseline survey, 23 percent had completed some college, and 8 percent had completed college. Five percent of study participants had full-time employment, and 11 percent had part-time employment at the time of the baseline survey. However, nearly two-thirds (65 percent) were unemployed and looking for work. Small percentages of participants were retired, students, homemakers, disabled or too ill to work, or had some other employment status. The majority of C2C study participants (51 percent) reported an individual income of less than $5,000 per year. Another 23 percent reported annual incomes between $5,000 and $20,000. Nine percent reported income between $20,000 and $40,000 per year. Fifteen percent of the C2C study participants did not provide an income level on the baseline survey.

Table 4.3. Demographic Information for C2C Study Participants (C2C group only), as of July 31, 2018 (n = 634)

	Number	Percentage
Gender		
Male	312	49
Female	308	49
Transgender woman or man, genderqueer, other gender identity	14	2
Age		
<18	23	4
18–24	253	40
25–30	98	15
31–40	112	18
Over 40	148	23
Ethnicity		
Hispanic/Latino	246	39
Race		
White/Caucasian	46	7
Black/African American	357	56
American Indian or Alaskan Native	14	2
Asian or Pacific Islander	8	1
Other	98	18
No response	111	18
Education level		
Less than high school	191	30
Completed high school with diploma or GED	217	34

	Number	Percentage
Some college	144	23
Completed college	51	8
Completed or some graduate or professional school	11	2
No response	20	3
Employment status		
Employed full-time	34	5
Employed part-time	70	11
Unemployed, looking for work	411	65
Student	55	9
Other (e.g., retired, homemaker, disabled)	37	6
No response	27	4
Individual Income level		
Less than $5,000	325	51
$5,000–10,000	78	12
$10,001–20,000	70	11
$20,001–30,000	32	5
$30,001–40,000	23	4
More than $40,000	13	2
No response	93	15

NOTE: In categories with fewer than five cases, we combined that category with another.

Baseline Survey

The eligibility screener included measures of five common mental health conditions. For baseline purposes, we stratified the C2C sample according to the symptom thresholds recommended by the publishers or in the literature, as they are more commonly used (Table 4.4). Among those who joined the C2C impact evaluation, over one-fifth (22 percent) reported depressive symptoms in the moderate to severe range, and an additional 19 percent reported mild depressive symptoms. Close to one-third (30 percent) reported moderate to severe anxiety. Thirty percent of C2C study participants scored higher than the suggested cut score on the measure of PTSD symptoms. For alcohol abuse, 13 percent reported alcohol use that indicated alcohol dependence, while an additional 10 percent reported harmful or hazardous drinking behavior. For substance abuse, 12 percent reported severe or substantial substance abuse whereas 16 percent reported behavior that indicated an intermediate level of substance abuse. Overall, 25 percent of participants in the C2C group reported symptoms in the moderate to severe range for only one condition, while 38 percent reported symptoms in the moderate to severe range for two conditions or more.

Table 4.4. Baseline Screening Information for C2C Study Participants (C2C group only), as of July 31, 2018 (*n* = 634)

	Number	Percentage
Depression (PHQ-8)		
None–Minimal depression	376	59
Mild depression	122	19
Moderate depression	83	13
Moderately severe depression	37	6
Severe depression	16	3
Anxiety (GAD-7)		
Mild	448	71
Moderate	105	17
Severe	81	13
PTSD		
≥cut score of 33	187	30
Alcohol abuse		
None	486	77
Harmful or hazardous drinking	64	10
Alcohol dependence	82	13
Substance abuse		
None	210	33
Low	247	39
Intermediate	104	16
Substantial	50	8
Severe	23	4

The baseline survey also asked participants about potential barriers to seeking mental health care (Table 4.5). Some of the most frequently cited barriers related to participants' views of their problems, with 73 percent wanting to solve the problem on their own and 59 percent believing the problem would resolve itself. About two-thirds of respondents indicated that their dislike of talking about issues (64 percent) and concerns about available treatment (60 percent) created barriers to seeking mental health care. The average number of barriers reported across all C2C study participants was 12.7 (of a possible a range of 0 to 30). Nearly one-fifth (19 percent) reported more than 20 barriers.

Table 4.5. Baseline Barriers to Seeking Professional Care for a Mental Health Problem Among C2C Study Participants (C2C group only), as of July 31, 2018 (*n* = 634)

Issue	Percentage Endorsed
Wanting to solve the problem on my own	73
Dislike of talking about my feelings, emotions or thoughts	64
Concerns about the treatments available (e.g., medication side effects)	60
Thinking the problem would get better by itself	59
Not being able to afford the costs	54
Thinking I did not have a problem	49
Feeing embarrassed or ashamed (S)	49
Thinking that professional care probably would not help	48
Concern that I might be seen as weak for having a mental health problem (S)	47
Concern that it might harm my chances when applying for jobs (S)	46
Concern about what my family might think, say, do or feel (S)	46
Being unsure where to go to get professional care	45
Concern that people might not take me seriously if they found out I was having professional care (S)	44
Concern that I might be seen as "crazy" (S)	44
Not wanting a mental health problem to be on my medical records (S)	43
Preferring to get alternative forms of care (e.g., traditional/religious healing, alternative/complementary therapies)	42
Preferring to get help from family or friends	42
Having no one who could help me get professional care	38
Difficulty taking time off work	38
Problems with transport or travelling to appointments	37
Concern that people I know might find out (S)	37
Concern about what my friends might think, say or do (S)	34
Being too unwell to ask for help	33
Concern about what people at work might think, say or do (S)	32
Having had previous bad experiences with professional care for mental health	31
Professionals from my own ethnic or cultural group not being available	26
Concern that I might be seen as a bad parent (S)	25
Concern that my children may be taken into care or that I may lose access or custody without my agreement (S)	21
Having problems with childcare while I receive professional care	17

NOTE: (S) indicates a stigma-related barrier.

The baseline survey also asked C2C study participants about their attitudes toward seeking professional help (Table 4.6). Overall, attitudes about professional help were mixed. A large majority of participants (79 percent) agreed that they would want to get psychological help if their worries continued for a long period of time. Participants also strongly endorsed other positive attitudes toward professional help, including being confident that psychotherapy would help for a serious emotional crisis (77 percent), and indicating that they might want counseling in the future (72 percent). Yet respondents also agreed with statements reflecting more negative attitudes toward professional help. For example, 68 percent of participants agreed that talking with a psychologist was not a good way to resolve emotional issues, and 61 percent agreed that personal and emotional troubles were likely to work out on their own.

Table 4.6. Attitudes Toward Seeking Professional Help Among C2C Study Participants (C2C group only), as of July 31, 2018 (n=634)

	Agree or Partly Agree (%)
Positive Attitude	
I would want to get psychological help if I were worried or upset for a long period of time.	79
If I were experiencing a serious emotional crisis at this point in my life, I would be confident that I could find relief in psychotherapy.	77
I might want to have psychological counseling in the future.	72
A person with an emotional problem is not likely to solve it alone; he or she is likely to solve it with professional help.	69
If I believed I was having a mental breakdown, my first inclination would be to get professional attention.	68
Negative Attitude	
The idea of talking about problems with a psychologist strikes me as a poor way to get rid of emotional conflicts.	68
Personal and emotional troubles, like many things, tend to work out by themselves.	61
Considering the time and expense involved in psychotherapy, it would have doubtful value for a person like me.	59
A person should work out his or her own problems; getting psychological counseling would be a last resort.	58
There is something admirable in the attitude of a person who is willing to cope with his or her conflicts and fears without resorting to professional help.	39

Finally, the baseline survey asked C2C study participants about their lifetime mental health service utilization (Table 4.7). Substantial proportions of participants had accessed each form of care. Over one-quarter (28 percent) had stayed overnight in a hospital for emotional, mental health, alcohol, or drug problems at some point. Furthermore, in the past six months, 11 percent had stayed overnight in a residential treatment program for alcohol or drug problems, with a range of one to 247 nights and an average of nearly 100 nights (i.e., more than three months). A substantial minority (37 percent) had gone to a hospital emergency room or an urgent care facility in the past six months for any health reason, with a range of one to 30 visits and an average of about three visits. One-third of C2C study participants had gone to a mental health provider in the past six months, with a range of one to 300 visits and an average of 15 visits. C2C study participants had also sought out other mental health services and supports in the past six months, including religious institutions (23 percent), substance abuse agencies (15 percent), support groups (13 percent), and community centers (14 percent). Eight percent had called a hotline for emotional, alcohol abuse, or substance abuse issues within the past six months.

Table 4.7. Mental Health Service Utilization Among C2C Study Participants (C2C group only), as of July 31, 2018 (*n* = 634)

Item	Number	Percentage
Have you ever stayed overnight in a hospital for emotional, mental health, alcohol or drug problems?	178	28
In the last 6 months, did you stay overnight in a residential treatment program for alcohol or drug problems?	65	11
In the last 6 months, did you go to a hospital emergency room or an urgent care facility for any health reason?	236	37
In the last 6 months, did you go to any mental health provider, including psychiatrists, psychologists, social workers, psychiatric nurses, or counselors?	205	33
Did you go to any religious or spiritual places such as a church, mosque, temple, or synagogue for emotional, mental health, alcohol or drug problems?	144	23
Did you go to any substance abuse agencies that have programs for people with drug or alcohol use problems or attend any self-help meetings such as Alcoholics Anonymous, Cocaine Anonymous, or Narcotics Anonymous?	92	15
Did you attend any self-help or family support groups for people with emotional or mental health problems?	82	13
Did you go to any parks and recreation or community centers for emotional, mental health, alcohol or drug problems?	91	14
Did you call a hotline for problems with your emotions or nerves, mental, alcohol, or drug problems?	49	8

Conclusions

As of July 2018, a total of 1,234 participants from 23 CBOs (13 C2C and ten comparison) had been screened for the impact evaluation. In this chapter, we provided a snapshot of data from mid-way through data collection, focusing on the C2C group (i.e., excluding data from the comparison group) to avoid premature conclusions about group differences. The study participants from C2C CBOs (634 individuals) were mostly over 18 years of age, were from ethnic minority backgrounds, and reported low incomes. Rates of moderate- to severe-level mental health concerns were similar to or higher than rates of mental health problems reported in the general population (Brody, Pratt, and Hughes, 2018). C2C participants endorsed a variety of barriers and a mix of positive and negative attitudes about seeking mental health care, suggesting that, despite relatively high rates of mental health concerns, many C2C clients were ambivalent about seeking care. A substantial proportion of the sampled participants had sought some form of help—including inpatient or residential behavioral health services—in the past. Although it is too early to draw any firm conclusions or make interpretations about the data from this partial sample alone, the impact evaluation analyses in the final report will pay close attention to these issues.

5. Summary of Interim Report

In this chapter, we summarize the interim evaluation findings, organized by evaluation component (implementation and impact; no cost findings are presented). We also summarize the evaluation's limitations, as they are important to consider when interpreting findings. No recommendations are made from these partial, preliminary data. The final report, to be made available in 2020, will include recommendations.

Implementation Evaluation Interim Conclusions

The freedom and flexibility of C2C allowed CBOs to adapt the program to their specific needs and infrastructure. But the variability in implementation options also presented challenges, particularly in the first year of the project, as CBOs pursued their individual plans. A number of early observations can be made:

- **CBO and MHP roles:** CBOs and MHPs had to sort out their respective roles early in implementation, including how and when to communicate about training, coaching, or client referrals, as well as how to gain familiarity with client populations and cultures. Most agreed, though, that efforts to learn about one another's organizational cultures and systems and to build opportunities for collaboration and communication into the C2C program infrastructure were helpful in fostering more effective working relationships.
- **Training:** In all cases, MHPs and CBOs worked collaboratively to develop and implement trainings for CBO staff. Efforts to tailor these trainings to best meet staff needs, and to incorporate feedback from CBO staff members, were seen as helpful in improving both staff buy-in and trainees' perceived value of training sessions— particularly in cases where the MHP did not have the initial capacity for training or supervision in one or more of the modalities (e.g., MI).
- **Coaching and Supervision:** CBOs placed increased emphasis on coaching and supervision practice in year 2. Most organizations were still developing—or in the early stages of implementing—coaching and supervision practices at the time of data collection.
- **Staff readiness:** In the annual staff survey, many staff endorsed confidence in using the C2C skills with clients. There was some indication that staff felt more comfortable with MHFA, MI, and screening than with psychoeducation. The structure and support of the MI Institute and formal MHFA trainings may have helped with staff familiarity with those skills. Most staff completing surveys also endorsed feeling comfortable talking about mental health issues with clients and noted that they had access to appropriate resources to help clients experiencing a mental health problem. In interviews, some CBO staff did report feeling uncomfortable talking with their clients about mental health issues, but they noted that the ability to practice using C2C skills and ongoing coaching and supervision helped tremendously. The majority of staff completing the survey felt supported by their organization and equipped to handle referrals.

- **Service delivery:** CBO staff members delivered C2C skills to thousands of clients, and the proportion of total CBO clients reached by C2C increased considerably in year 2 of implementation as sites began to implement all four core C2C skills. On average, CBO direct service staff reported spending more than eight hours per week delivering C2C skills and/or referring clients to mental health treatment.
- **Perceived impact:** C2C has been seen by key informants as driving a positive shift in organizational culture regarding mental health. Interviewees also reported witnessing direct benefits to staff mental health and coping with work stressors. Staff and clients reported benefits to clients, most notably with respect to reduced stigma toward mental health and increased comfort discussing mental health concerns with CBO staff. Several barriers to referring clients to treatment were noted, and both CBOs and MHPs have taken a number of steps to help mitigate these challenges and improve access to services for clients with mental health treatment needs.

Impact Evaluation Interim Conclusions

As of July 2018, a total of 1,234 participants from 23 CBOs (13 C2C and ten comparison) had been screened for the impact evaluation. About 85 percent of these individuals were eligible for the study based on scores on five mental health screeners (depression, anxiety, PTSD, and alcohol and drug abuse) that met the study's minimum threshold for eligibility, and 85 percent of eligible individuals completed baseline surveys. Demographics of the participants who are clients of C2C CBOs (634 individuals) indicate that clients largely reflected the target population, with most over 18 years of age and reporting low incomes (51 percent reported earning less than $5,000 per year). Most C2C participants were also from ethnic minority backgrounds (only 7 percent were White/Caucasian). Rates of moderate- to severe-level mental health concerns among C2C study participants ranged from 22 percent (for depression) to 30 percent (for PTSD) at baseline. These rates are similar to or higher than rates of mental health problems reported in the general population and suggest that a substantial proportion of C2C clients need mental health support. For example, in a national survey (National Health and Nutrition Examination Survey) that used the same depression screener (PHQ), approximately 8 percent of adults over age 20 screened positive for depression (Brody, Pratt, and Hughes, 2018).

In baseline surveys, C2C participants endorsed a range of barriers to seeking professional mental health care, with at least 60 percent reporting "wanting to solve the problem on my own," "dislike of talking about my feelings, emotions or thoughts," and "concerns about the treatments available (e.g., medication side effects)" as barriers. Participants also endorsed a mix of positive and negative attitudes about seeking mental health care, suggesting that, despite relatively high rates of mental health concerns, many C2C clients may be ambivalent about seeking care. This ambivalence is interesting, given that a substantial proportion of the sample had received formal mental health care previously. For example, 28 percent of the sample had received inpatient care for mental health problems in their lifetime.

It is too early to draw conclusions or make interpretations about these data based on this partial sample. Some of the CBOs that contributed the most participants to the current sample are also organizations that serve populations who are particularly likely to have experience with the formal mental health system (e.g., formerly incarcerated individuals). Data collection began at each CBO at a different point in time, and we did not attempt to compare the C2C group to the comparison group for the purposes of this interim report. Thus, we avoid drawing any firm conclusions about the extent to which the sample described here is representative of low-income communities in New York City or elsewhere. The impact evaluation analyses in the final report (to be delivered in 2020) will utilize the full sample, from both C2C and comparison groups, to make more concrete observations.

Limitations

It is important to consider the evaluation's limitations when interpreting its findings. As noted throughout the report, the data used for the implementation evaluation come from a mix of sources, including a staff survey and site visits that were conducted one year prior to this report, at a time when CBOs were in an early stage of implementation. Thus, the findings described here cannot fully depict the C2C implementation process. In addition, the implementation processes, challenges, and successes described here are based on information from the 15 CBOs that are currently participating in the program. While some of the lessons learned may be generalizable to other organizations, some implementation experiences likely are unique, hinging on individual CBO characteristics, the current policy and funding environment, and the novelty of the C2C program. Other CBOs seeking to replicate the program may encounter additional challenges (or successes). In the final report, to be released in 2020, we will be positioned to more fully describe C2C implementation across CBOs, and this information should help other organizations to design and/or plan C2C-like implementation in the future.

Similarly, the impact evaluation data come from the early or mid-stage of data collection. We caution readers that the data reported in Chapter 4 are only a snapshot of a single point in time and should not be considered representative of the final sample. Since enrollment in the impact evaluation's client survey will continue through March 2019, the sample characteristics and baseline data will likely change. We do not yet have follow-up data to report from the impact evaluation, so we cannot speak to how symptoms may be fluctuating over time and in response to receipt of C2C programming.

Readers should also note that the site visit and staff and client survey data are all based on self-report, and that the data come from a subsample of individuals who volunteered to participate in those portions of the evaluation. Administrative data from CBOs and New York City and state agencies will be triangulated with these data for the final report analyses, but such data were not ready for use at the time of this interim report. Finally, we also remind readers that we excluded individuals who did not report mental health symptoms on the five screeners. Thus, findings may not be generalizable to all staff or clients who participated in the C2C program overall.

Next Steps

At the time of writing, CBOs and MHPs are moving beyond the early implementation and training stages of the program and are focusing their efforts on full program implementation. Over the next two years, we will continue to evaluate C2C implementation, impact, and cost. Implementation and cost evaluation data collection, including staff surveys, key informant interviews, and CBO program data, will continue through 2019. Impact study participant enrollment at both C2C and comparison CBO sites will continue through March 2019, with follow-up assessments ending in March 2020. A final report will be made available in 2020.

Appendix A. Methods and Measures

This appendix describes the methods used in the C2C implementation, impact, and cost evaluations in further detail. We note measures and methods that were not used in the interim report where applicable.

Implementation Evaluation

Key Informant Interviews and Focus Groups

We conducted in-person site visits with the 15 CBOs and their MHP partners from June to August 2017 and held separate key informant interviews/focus groups with leadership, staff, and clients. We developed separate interview guides for CBO leadership, MHP leadership, CBO staff, and CBO clients to collect qualitative information on a range of topics, including, but not limited to,

- implementation challenges and areas for improvement
- implementation facilitators and successes
- experiences with training on C2C supports
- delivery of C2C supports to clients
- collaboration between CBOs and their MHPs
- client engagement in C2C and referrals to MHPs
- client perspectives on C2C experience/quality/satisfaction.

During the 2017 site visits, researchers visited all 15 CBOs and interviewed 35 CBO leaders (e.g., CBO executive directors, CBO C2C program directors), 29 MHP leaders (e.g., MHP clinical directors, MHP counselors), 80 participating CBO frontline staff (e.g., trained in and providing C2C supports to CBO clients), and 38 CBO clients who were offered and/or received C2C supports. Leadership and frontline staff interviewees included organizational leaders and program managers, psychologists, social workers, client intake specialists, case managers, job counselors, and life skills instructors, among others. These individuals were involved in roles such as coordination and oversight of C2C supports within the CBO, supervision and training of CBO staff, and direct delivery of C2C supports to clients.

Interviews were mainly conducted in the form of focus groups, with multiple interviewees attending per session. This format was chosen to reduce the burden for participating interviewees, facilitate scheduling during one-day or two-day site visits, and limit disruption to regular programming at CBOs and MHPs. Some interviews with CBO leads and clients were conducted with a single interviewee because of availability and/or interviewee preferences. After obtaining consent from each interviewee, the interviews were audio recorded. If an interviewee consented to participate in the interview but declined to be audio recorded, the interview was not audio recorded. Interviews were conducted by two research staff: One led the interview, while a second captured as much of the conversation as possible in written notes in real time; audio recordings were used to confirm accuracy and completeness of real-time notes.

Annual Staff Survey

From May to September 2017, an online survey was administered to all CBO staff who were trained in at least one of the four C2C supports (i.e., screening, MI, MHFA, psychoeducation). The purpose of the survey was to collect quantitative data on

- the educational and occupational backgrounds of CBO staff participating in C2C
- experiences with C2C training and supervision
- attitudes toward mental health, including mental health stigma
- organizational climate and access to resources
- helping behaviors toward clients with mental health issues
- level of confidence in ability to deliver C2C supports.

During the survey time frame, CBOs provided researchers with contact information for 477 staff members who had completed training in at least one of the C2C supports. These individuals were invited by email to complete an online survey. Of these, 58 individuals were ineligible for the survey or could not be contacted (i.e., had not received training in C2C; no longer worked at the organization; email message bounced back), and four individuals declined consent to participate. A total of 140 CBO staff members responded to the survey, for a response rate of 34 percent. Approximately half (52 percent) of respondents were direct service providers (e.g., counselors, educators, service coordinators); 27 percent were leadership, management, or supervisors; and 21 percent were administrative or other staff (e.g., security, receptionist). Most of the sample (62 percent) had been involved with the organization for between one and five years; 15 percent had been with the organization for less than one year, and 23 percent had been involved for more than five years.

Demographics

These questions include age, gender identity, race/ethnicity, language, education/degree, mental health, and substance use.

Background

These questions include CBO/organization, occupation/job role, experience in the industry (less than five years, five to ten years, more than ten years), and job details (full-time paid employee, part-time paid employee, unpaid employee, intern).

Training and Use of Skills

Our scale includes 14 items covering the following domains:

- training in modalities (behavioral health screening, psychoeducation, MI, MHFA)

- training duration (how many total hours of training for each of the C2C modalities)
- manual or protocol (receipt of a written training manual or protocol)
- booster sessions/coaching (receipt of booster sessions, supervision or coaching in C2C modalities after initial training; type of coaching/supervision)
- satisfaction with training (satisfied with training in C2C modalities; satisfied with supervision; training in C2C modalities has improved my ability to help my clients with mental health problems; I could use additional training, coaching, and/or supervision in C2C mental health modalities)
- use of skills (with what proportion of clients have you used *any* of the C2C modalities)
- delivery of C2C modalities (how often do you provide screening, psychoeducation, MHFA, MI)
- confidence to administer C2C modalities. How confident are you in your ability to

  - administer behavioral health screening to clients?
  - provide psychoeducation to clients?
  - provide mental health first aid to clients?
  - provide motivational interviewing to clients?

Time Allocated to C2C

These six items assess amount of time spent delivering C2C mental health supports to clients, number of separate occasions (e.g., discrete service delivery sessions) in which staff delivered C2C supports to clients, and amount of time spent with clients during a typical C2C service delivery session.

Time Allocated to C2C

- During the past year, how many hours per week did you typically work at this job?
- Out of the past 12 months, how many months did you work on the C2C program?
- In a typical week in the past month, how many hours did you spend working on C2C program activities?

Time Allocated to Specific C2C Services

- In a typical week in the past month, how did you allocate your time spent on C2C activities?

  - delivering C2C modalities to clients (behavioral health screening, MI, MHFA, psychoeducation)
  - referring C2C clients to behavioral health providers
  - participation in technical assistance from the RAND Corporation /NYU McSilver, including email, phone, webinar, or in-person interactions with the RAND Corporation or NYU McSilver staff
  - receiving or giving training on C2C modalities and referrals for C2C clients
  - data collection and reporting to Mayor's Fund or C2C evaluator (RAND Corporation/NYU McSilver)
  - supervising CBO staff on C2C program, coordinating with the mental health provider partner, and ensuring that the C2C program operates as expected

- clinical supervision of C2C modality delivery
- other activity.

Occasions per Modality Service Delivery

- If you delivered behavioral health services or made referrals in a typical week of the past month, on how many separate occasions did you deliver one or more of the following behavioral health services?

    - behavioral health screening
    - MI
    - MHFA
    - psychoeducation
    - mental health and/or substance use counseling
    - coping skills or stress management training
    - case management for mental health/substance use treatment
    - referring clients to behavioral health providers
    - other.

Time per Occasion of Modality Service Delivery

- If you delivered behavioral health services or made referrals in a typical week in the past month, how much time (in minutes) did you spend on delivering one or more of the following behavioral health services on a typical occasion?

    - behavioral health screening
    - MI
    - MHFA
    - psychoeducation
    - mental health and/or substance use counseling
    - coping skills or stress management training
    - case management for mental health/substance use treatment
    - referring clients to behavioral health providers
    - other.

[not included in interim report] **Stigma and Staff Blame.** Twelve stigma survey questions were adapted from the devaluation-discrimination measures from Link et al.'s (1989) modified labeling theory. These items assess the extent to which respondents believe that most people will devalue or discriminate against a person with a history of psychiatric treatment. Two items assess blame (beliefs about whether staff member would be blamed or held responsible if a client harmed himself/herself/others) were adapted from Ramchand et al.'s (2015) survey assessing key domains of gatekeeper behavior among persons who identify service members at risk of suicide and refer them to treatment. Items were answered with a six-point Likert scale from 1 (strongly disagree) to 6 (strongly agree).

Stigma

1. Most people would willingly accept someone with history of behavioral health problems as a close friend.
2. Most people believe that someone with history of behavioral health problems is just as intelligent as the average person.
3. Most people believe that someone with history of behavioral health problems is just as trustworthy as the average citizen.
4. Most people would accept someone with history of behavioral health problems as a teacher of young children in a public school.
5. Most people feel that entering a treatment facility of behavioral health problems is a sign of personal failure.
6. Most people would not hire someone with a history of behavioral health problems to take care of their children, even if he or she has been in recovery for some time.
7. Most people think less of someone with a history of behavioral health problems.
8. Most employers will hire someone with a history of behavioral health problems if he or she is qualified for the job.
9. Most employers will pass over the application of someone with a history of behavioral health problems in favor or another applicant.
10. Most people in my community would treat someone with a history of behavioral health problems just as they would treat anyone.
11. Most young people would be reluctant to date someone with a history of behavioral health problems.
12. Once they know a person has a history of behavioral health problems, most people will take his or her opinions less seriously.

Blame

1. If I talked to a client about their thoughts about harming himself/herself or harming others, and someone was later harmed, I would be held responsible.
2. If one of my clients harms himself/herself or others, I would be held responsible regardless of whether I spoke to him/her or not.

[not included in interim report] **Mental Health Knowledge and Attitudes.** Twelve items were adapted from the Mental Health Knowledge Schedule (Evans-Lacko et al., 2010). This scale assesses stigma-related mental health knowledge among the general public. Items were answered with a five-point Likert scale from 1 (strongly disagree) to 5 (strongly agree).

1. Most people with behavioral health problems want to have paid employment.
2. If a friend had a behavioral health problem, I know what advice to give them to get professional help.
3. Medication can be an effective treatment for people with behavioral health problems.
4. Psychotherapy (for example, talking therapy or counseling) can be an effective treatment for people with behavioral health problems.
5. People with severe behavioral health problems can fully recover.
6. Most people with behavioral health problems go to a health care professional to get help
7. Depression is a mental illness.
8. Stress is a mental illness.

9. Schizophrenia is a mental illness.
10. Bipolar disorder (manic depression) is a mental illness.
11. Drug addiction is a mental illness.
12. Grief is a mental illness.

[Organizational Climate items not included in interim report] **Organizational Climate and Support.** Twenty-five survey items in three domains: access to resources, efficacy, and organizational climate. The access to resources and efficacy items were adapted from the Survey of Knowledge, Attitudes, and Gatekeeper Behaviors for Suicide Prevention in Schools (Wyman et al., 2008; Tompkins and Witt, 2009). Organizational climate questions were adapted from Lehman, Greener, and Simpson (2002). Access to resources and efficacy items were answered with a five-point Likert scale from 1 (strongly disagree) to 6 (strongly agree); organizational climate items were answered with a five-point Likert scale from 1 (strongly disagree) to 5 (strongly agree).

Access to Resources

1. I have easy access to the educational or resource materials I need to learn about behavioral health.
2. My organization has access to an adequate number of resources or people to whom I could refer clients experiencing behavioral health difficulties.
3. I can identify the places or people where I should refer clients experiencing behavioral health difficulties.

Efficacy

1. My organization encourages me to ask clients about behavioral health difficulties
2. I feel comfortable discussing behavioral health issues with clients
3. I am aware of the warning signs of behavioral health problems
4. I can recognize clients experiencing behavioral health difficulties by the way they behave
5. My training to assist clients who are experiencing behavioral health issues is insufficient
6. I don't have the necessary skills to discuss behavioral health issues with clients
7. I know most clients well enough to question them about behavioral health issues

Organizational Climate

1. Ideas and suggestions from staff get fair consideration by program management.
2. The formal and informal communication channels here work very well.
3. Program staff are always kept well informed.
4. More open discussions about program issues are needed here.
5. Staff members always feel free to ask questions and express concerns in this program.
6. Some staff get confused about the main goals for this program.
7. Program staff understand how this program fits as part of the treatment system in your community.
8. Your duties are clearly related to the goals of this program.
9. This program operates with clear goals and objectives.
10. Management here has a clear plan for this program.

11. You are under too many pressures to do your job effectively.
12. Staff members often show signs of stress and strain.
13. The heavy workload here reduces program effectiveness.
14. Staff frustration is common here.
15. Frequent staff turnover is a problem for this program.

Staff Behaviors and Perceptions. Twenty items assess staff intervention behaviors, important factors in referral decisions, and perceptions of clients' comfort with discussing mental health–related issues. The items assessing staff intervention behaviors were adapted from a survey of knowledge, attitudes, and gatekeeper behaviors for suicide prevention in schools. This survey was used to evaluate a gatekeeper training for university resident advisers aiming to improve detection and referral of at-risk students (Tompkins and Witt, 2009; Shaffer et al., 1991). Items were answered with a five-point Likert scale from 1 (never) to 5 (always), with 0 = not applicable. For important factors in referral decisions, items were answered with a six-point Likert scale from 1 (not at all important) to 6 (very much important) and were developed by the RAND evaluation team. Items assessing staff perceptions of clients' comfort in discussing behavioral health-related concerns (also developed by the RAND evaluation team) were answered with a five-point Likert scale from 1 (strongly disagree) to 5 (strongly agree).

Intervention Behaviors

When you suspect of know a client is experiencing behavioral health issues, how often do you:

1. ask the client about behavioral health issues
2. convince the client to seek help
3. escort a client to a counselor or other resource
4. get advice from a co-worker
5. keep it a secret
6. left him/her alone until he/she feels better
7. refer them to a behavioral health care provider (e.g., a psychologist)
8. provide the client with information (e.g., how to get help for behavioral health issues; education about behavioral health)
9. spend time listening to the client
10. talk to a supervisor about the client
11. other.

Important Factors in Referral Decisions.

Please rate how important each of the following factors are to you in deciding where to refer a client for behavioral health services:

1. confidentiality
2. convenience
3. length of time expected to get an appointment
4. policies of your organization
5. quality of care

6. other

Client Comfort

Please rate how much you agree or disagree with the following statements:

1. My clients do or would feel comfortable talking about their behavioral health issues with me.
2. My clients do or would feel comfortable accepting a referral to a behavioral health provider inside of my organization.
3. My clients do or would feel comfortable accepting a referral to a behavioral health provider outside of my organization (i.e., an external referral).

CBO Quarterly Report Data

CBOs submitted quarterly report data to the C2C collaborative once per quarter between March 2016 and March 2018. Reports included both qualitative descriptions of key challenges and successes, as well as aggregate data on a range of implementation metrics, including staff training, supervision and coaching activities, delivery of C2C supports to clients, and client referrals (Table A.1). Reports were reviewed for completeness and accuracy by the C2C Collaborative as well as the RAND evaluation team. CBOs worked closely with the C2C Collaborative to resolve any errors in data entry.

Table A.1. Quarterly Progress Report Data Elements

Evaluation Area	Data Element
Staff training	<ul><li>Number of CBO staff</li><li>Number of staff trained in each modality</li><li>Number of staff trained in all four modalities</li><li>Number of CBO supervisors</li><li>Number of supervisors trained</li><li>Number of supervisors trained in each modality</li><li>Number of supervisors trained in all four modalities</li><li>Total (staff and supervisors) trained for the first time</li></ul>
Staff coaching	<ul><li>Number of staff who received continuous coaching and supervision (MI)</li><li>Number of staff who received continuous coaching and supervision (psychoeducation, screening and referral, or MHFA)</li><li>Number of supervisors who received continuous coaching and supervision (MI)</li><li>Number of supervisors who received continuous coaching and supervision (psychoeducation, screening and referral, or mhfa)</li><li>Total (staff and supervisors) who received continuous coaching and supervision</li><li>Number of training hours provided by MHP</li><li>Number of coaching and supervision hours provided by MHP</li></ul>
Client receipt of services	<ul><li>Number of program participants</li><li>Number of new C2C participants</li><li>Number of program participants who received a C2C modality</li><li>Number of program participants who received screening</li><li>Number of program participants who screened positive</li><li>Number of program participants who received psychoeducation</li><li>Number of program participants who were referred to the MHP partner</li><li>Number of program participants who were referred to an external mental or behavioral health provider</li><li>Number of participants who screened positive and were referred to the MHP or an external provider</li><li>Number of program participants who completed referral at the MHP partner</li><li>Number of program participants who completed referral at the external provider</li></ul>
Client demographics	<ul><li>Gender</li><li>Age</li><li>Race/ethnicity</li><li>Country of origin</li></ul>

[not included in interim report] Core Component Fidelity Checklists: Annual C2C Supervisor and RAND Evaluator Observations of CBO Staff Delivering C2C Modalities

C2C Supervisor Ratings

CBO and MHP supervisors conduct supervisory sessions with CBO staff and, when possible, direct observations of CBO staff delivering C2C mental health supports as part of the C2C program. Supervisors use information obtained from regular supervisory activities to complete annual ratings of CBO modality adherence using core component fidelity checklists. For instances in which supervisors are unable to directly observe C2C modality delivery (e.g., because of the spontaneous, ad hoc nature of delivering modalities such as MHFA and MI), supervisors document this and assess fidelity based on role-play activities and the staff member's self-report of an episode in which he or she delivered that modality.

RAND Evaluator Ratings

We conduct direct observations of CBO staff during delivery of C2C modalities to clients within the annual site visits. Observations are limited to group activities (e.g., group psychoeducation sessions) to minimize risk to staff and clients and mitigate disruption to service provision. Participation in direct observations is voluntary, and CBO staff members and clients are asked to provide consent for their participation; individuals who decline to consent are not subject to any penalty.

Checklists

We developed checklists in consultation with the Mayor's Fund and Department of Health and Mental Hygiene. Raters use the core fidelity checklist tools developed for each modality to assess fidelity with delivering C2C treatments. Ratings are aggregated to examine fidelity with C2C modalities at the CBO level. As the fidelity checklists are comparable in structure and content for all CBOs, fidelity scores are compared across CBOs to examine differences across sites. Example metrics include percentage of fidelity checklists in which all items were checked as complete, number of times each C2C modality observed, and number of CBO staff observed.

The checklist includes the following elements:

For Each C2C Support

- was staff member trained—if so, when
- staff skill level in delivering modality (unacceptable, poor, fair, average, good, very good/excellent)
- level of confidence in staff member's skill level (not at all confident, somewhat confidence, very confident)

Use of Core Components

Screening: Did staff complete this component? (Yes, No, Don't know)

- introduced the screening instrument
- administered the screening instrument
- scored the screening instrument
- reviewed results of the screening with the participant
- assisted the client in interpreting the meaning of these results
- followed the protocol established by your workplace for managing participants after screening.

Psychoeducation: Did staff complete this component? (Yes, No, Don't know)

- engaged the participant in a guided, structured discussion and provided detailed information on a specific behavioral health-related topic in a one-on-one or group context

- psychoeducation provided to the participant was curriculum-based and supported by data
- offered to provide the participants with additional resources relevant to the content of psychoeducation.

Mental Health First Aid: Did staff complete this component? (Yes, No, Don't know)

- identified that a participant was experiencing signs/symptoms of a mental health or substance use problem and engaged participant in a discussion about mental health concerns
- assessed for risk of suicide or harm
- listened nonjudgmentally
- gave reassurance and information about mental health
- encouraged appropriate professional help
- encouraged self-help and other support strategies.

Motivational Interviewing: Did staff complete this component? (Yes, No, Don't know)

- engaged the client in a focused discussion about a specific topic related to behavior change
- assisted the client in resolving ambivalence or uncertainty about change
- provided unsolicited advice, directions, or feedback to the client about how the client should change
- utilized specific MI tools or strategies to facilitate the discussion about behavior change, including but not limited to rolling with resistance, OARS, highlighting and developing discrepancies. eliciting "change talk," "values" sort, readiness rulers, assess readiness to, confidence in, and importance for change, support client self-efficacy to change
- directly confronted the client or argued with the client about the client's need to change
- adhered to the style and "spirit" of MI during discussion about change (e.g., nonjudgmental, collaborative, non-confrontational, and person-centered approach).

[not included in interim report] CBO Program Data

CBOs will submit program data on C2C service delivery and staff participation in C2C training and supervision activities.

Individual-Level De-Identified CBO Program Data for Clients

When data are available, each C2C CBO will submit the following de-identified individual-level program data for clients:

- demographics (e.g., age range, race/ethnicity, gender, country of origin, education, employment status)
- dates and frequency C2C services were offered and received
- dates referrals were offered and accepted
- referral follow-through/appointment attended
- dates that CBO services were completed for the client (i.e., job placement, GED obtained, housing status/placement).

Individual-Level CBO Staff Data

C2C CBOs will submit individual-level staff data (when available) on dates and length of sessions in which staff delivered C2C modalities, participated in C2C trainings, and received or provided C2C coaching and supervision.

Impact Evaluation

Client Survey Screening Measures

PHQ-8. The PHQ-8 is an eight-item self-report measure of current depression that asks respondents to indicate how often they have been bothered by each symptom of depression in the previous two weeks (see Table A.2 for more details on this measure and others listed below). The measure can be used in clinical samples and in the general population. Items are coded 0 to 3, and scores are summed to generate a total score, ranging from 0 to 24, with higher scores indicating higher depressive symptoms. Scores greater than or equal to ten indicate moderate depression. C2C program participants are eligible for participation in the impact study if they report at least mild symptoms of depression, with a score greater than or equal to five. Prior research using the PHQ-8 provides evidence of good internal consistency, with Cronbach's alphas ranging from 0.86 to 0.89 and good sensitivity and specificity for identifying cases with diagnoses of major depressive disorder (Kroenke et al., 2009).

GAD-7. The GAD-7 is a seven-item self-report measure of current anxiety that asks respondents to indicate how often they have been bothered by each symptom of anxiety in the previous two weeks. Scores of zero to four are considered minimal, five to ten mild, ten to 14 moderate, and 15 to 21 severe. C2C program participants are eligible for participation in the impact study if they report a score greater than or equal to five. The measure has been used in a wide range of populations and can be used in clinical samples and in the general population to screen and monitor (over repeated assessments) for symptoms of anxiety. The GAD-7 has been demonstrated to have strong internal consistency ($\alpha = 0.89$) and good sensitivity and specificity for identifying cases with diagnosis of generalized anxiety disorder (Spitzer et al., 2006; Löwe et al., 2008).

PCL-5. The PCL-5 is a 20-item self-report measure of PTSD symptoms designed for use in primary care populations and has been used in a wide range of demographic groups among individuals ages 18 and older. Cut scores for predicting PTSD diagnostic status have not yet been established for the PCL-5, and range from 30 to 60 depending on the population, setting, and assessment goal (Blevins et al., 2015). A cut point of 33 is suggestive of PTSD diagnosis. C2C program participants are eligible for participation in the impact study if they report a score greater than or equal to 28. A provisional DSM-5 PTSD diagnosis may be obtained by considering items rated moderately or higher as symptoms endorsed and following the DSM-5 diagnostic rule (at least one B, one C, two D, and two E symptoms present) (Blevins et al.,

2015). Prior research shows that this measure demonstrates excellent internal consistency (α = 0.94), correlates highly with other scales of PTSD symptoms ($r > 0.84$), and has good sensitivity and specificity for identifying cases with PTSD (Blevins et al., 2015).

AUDIT-10. The AUDIT-10 is a ten-item self-report scale used to identify risky or harmful alcohol consumption as well as alcohol use disorders, and to assess the amount and frequency of alcohol intake, alcohol dependence, and problems related to alcohol consumption. Scores range from zero to 40. The cut-off point for potentially hazardous alcohol intake is eight, although the cut-off score may differ depending on the specific population (e.g., men and women have different cut-off points). C2C program participants are eligible for participation in the impact study if they report a score greater than or equal to eight. In prior research, the AUDIT-10 has been shown to have good sensitivity and specificity for identifying cases with alcohol use disorders (Berner et al., 2007; Babor et al., 1992).

DAST-10. The DAST-10 is a self-report measure of problematic substance use that is utilized for clinical screening and research. The ten-item instrument has been used in a wide variety of populations, including adolescents and adults in a range of demographic groups. Scores greater than or equal to three indicate moderate substance abuse. C2C program participants are eligible for participation in the impact study if they report a score greater than or equal to one. The DAST-10 has strong internal consistency (α = 0.74–0.92) and good test-retest reliability ($r = 0.71$), and correlates very highly with the longer DAST-20 instrument ($r = 0.98$). The scale also demonstrates good sensitivity and specificity for identifying cases with substance use/misuse disorders (Yudko, Lozhkina, and Fouts, 2007).

Table A.2. Client Survey Screening Measures

	Diagnostic Cutoff	Study Eligibility Cutoff
Depression	0–4 = minimal 5–9 = mild 10–14 = moderate 15–19 = moderately severe 20–24 = severe	PHQ-8≥5
Anxiety	0–9 = mild 10–14 = moderate ≥15 = severe	GAD-7≥5
PTSD	≥33 = provisional PTSD diagnosis	PCL-5≥28
Alcohol abuse	< 8 = none **Female**: 8–12 = harmful or hazardous ≥13 = alcohol dependence **Male**: 8–14 = harmful or hazardous ≥15 = alcohol dependence	AUDIT≥8
Substance abuse	0 = none 1–2 = low 3–5 = intermediate 6–8 = substantial 9–10 = severe	DAST-10≥1

Client Survey Assessment Measures

Barriers to Access to Care Evaluation (BACEv2). The BACEv2 has 30 items. It is used as a measure of a range of different barriers to accessing mental health care in community populations and can be used to assess change in barriers to care after the introduction of community interventions to increase care-seeking and service use. Prior research provides evidence of good test-retest reliability, and good convergent and construct validity (Clement et al., 2012).

Attitudes Toward Seeking Professional Psychological Help Scale – Short Form (ATSPPH-SF). The ATSPPH-SF is a self-report measure of attitudes toward seeking mental health treatment. The 12 items are each coded 0 to 3 (disagree–agree). Total scores range from zero to 30, with higher scores indicating more favorable treatment attitudes. The scale has strong internal consistency ($\alpha = 0.82$–0.84) and good test-retest reliability (Elhai, Schweinle, and Anderson, 2008).

Mental health service utilization questions from the National Survey on Drug Use and Health (NSDUH). The interviewer-administered NSDUH mental health service utilization questions have been used in a wide variety of populations in the United States (Substance Abuse and Mental Health Services Administration, 2003). Nine survey items assessing mental health service utilization were administered to C2C participants (Table 3.7).

[not included in interim report] **World Health Organization Quality of Life – BREF (WHOQOL-BREF).** The WHOQOL-BREF is a person-centered, multilingual instrument for

multidimensional assessment of quality of life. The scale assesses a broad range of quality of life facets in four domains: physical, psychological, social, and environmental. It can be self-administered and is designed for generic use as a multidimensional profile that can be compared across a wide range of populations (e.g., clinical and nonclinical samples, groups with different diseases and conditions). Prior research provides evidence of good internal consistency (α = 0.68–0.82) across four domains and good discriminant validity of sick and well respondents (Skevington, Lotfy, and O'Connell, 2004). The overall quality of life question was administered to C2C participants as one measure of functioning.

[not included in interim report] **World Health Organization Disability Assessment Schedule (WHODAS 2.0).** The WHODAS is a widely used measure of disability. The 12-item scale is intended for use in community samples and has been used across a range of different ethnic and cultural groups. The WHODAS has good test-retest reliability and convergent validity (Ustun et al., 2010).

[not included in interim report] **Kessler 6 (K-6).** The K-6 is a widely used measure of general distress. The scale has six items and has been validated in in primary care clinics, community mental health centers, and social welfare offices. Prior research shows that this measure demonstrates good test-retest reliability and convergent validity (Kessler et al., 2003).

[not included in interim report] **Trauma History Screen (THS).** The THS is a 13-item self-administered measure of trauma history that asks respondents to indicate whether and how many times they had experienced each event in their lifetime. The measure can be used in clinical samples and in the general population and has been used in a wide range of populations including those with low reading levels. This measure has been proven to have good test-retest reliability, construct validity, and convergent validity (Carlson et al., 2005).

[not included in interim report] **Stressful events questions from the Life Experiences Survey (LES).** The adapted LES is a seven-item self-administered measure of stressful experiences that asks respondents to indicate whether they have experienced each event in the past 12 months. The measure can be used in clinical samples and in the general population and has been used in a wide range of populations including urban, low-income ethnic minority populations. Test-retest reliability and convergent validity for the LES were reported as strong (Sarason, Johnson, and Siegel, 1978).

[not included in interim report] CBO Program Data

CBOs will submit program data on C2C service delivery for clients who consent to participate in the impact evaluation client survey.

Individual-level identifiable CBO program data for clients. When data are available, each C2C CBO will submit the following identifiable individual-level program data for clients: demographics (e.g., age range, race/ethnicity, gender, country of origin, education, employment status); dates/frequency C2C services were offered and received, dates referrals were offered and accepted, referral follow-through/appointment attended; dates that CBO services were completed for the client (i.e., job placement, GED obtained, housing status/placement).

[not included in interim report] Administrative Data from New York City and State

New York City and New York State agencies will share administrative data on specific data elements (e.g., Medicaid claims, emergency department visits, unemployment benefits, homeless shelter stays) for C2C program and comparison group participants who consent to participate in this aspect of the study. Currently, we are requesting administrative data from the following agencies and organizations:

- New York City Department of Corrections
- New York State Department of Corrections and Community Services
- New York State Department of Labor
- New York City Health and Hospitals Corporation
- New York City Human Resources Administration
- New York City Department of Homeless Services
- New York State Office of Medicaid
- New York City Housing Authority.

Cost Evaluation

No cost evaluation findings are included in the interim report. The cost evaluation is being conducted with data collected from the following sources: CBO financial reports, biannual cost surveys, annual non-labor expense reports, annual compensation reports, participant assessments from the individuals who are enrolled in the Impact Evaluation, and administrative data from the government agencies of New York City and New York State (see Table A.3 for the measures included).

Table A.3. Cost Evaluation Measures

Measure Name	Definition
Average project cost per CBO	The average of total expenditures spent on the C2C program per CBO (i.e. C2C project cost divided by number of CBOs).
Average cost per CBO per quarter	The average of total expenditures in each quarter, for all quarters in which CBOs incurred costs. The number of CBOs incurring costs varies by quarter; in these instances, total C2C project cost per quarter is divided by only the number of CBOs that incurred costs.
Annualized project cost per CBO	Average cost per CBO per year (i.e. average cost per CBO per quarter multiplied by four quarters).
Total cost	Sum of expenditures spent by each CBO on labor, contracted services, other direct costs, and indirect costs (as detailed below).
Labor cost	Expenditures on salaries and fringe benefits.
Contracted services cost	Payments that CBOs make via a contract, including MHP providers and other consultants.

Measure Name	Definition
Other direct cost	Expenditures on other costs, including rent, utilities, network or computing costs, equipment, supplies, travel, training, and criminal history checks.
Indirect costs	Cost of overhead expenditures (typically a percentage of total labor and other direct costs).
Average cost per client served	The average of total expenditures spent per client served by CBOs (i.e., total cost/number of clients served). Total number of clients served only includes the sum of clients served in quarters for which CBO expenditures were recorded.

References

Aarons, G. A., M. Hurlburt, and S. M. Horwitz, "Advancing a Conceptual Model of Evidence-Based Practice Implementation in Public Service Sectors," *Administration and Policy in Mental Health*, Vol. 38, No. 1, 2011, pp. 4–23.

Acri, M., S. Frank, S. S. Olin, G. Burton, J. L. Ball, J. Weaver, and K. E. Hoagwood, "Examining the Feasibility and Acceptability of a Screening and Outreach Model Developed for a Peer Workforce," *Journal of Child and Family Studies*, Vol. 24, No. 2, 2015, pp. 341–350.

Acri, M., S. S. Olin, G. Burton, R. J. Herman, and K. E. Hoagwood, "Innovations in the Identification and Referral of Mothers at Risk for Depression: Development of a Peer-to-Peer Model," *Journal of Child and Family Studies*, Vol. 23, No. 5, 2014, pp. 837–843.

Aitken, C., D. Wain, D. I. Lubman, L. Hides, and M. Hellard, "Mental Health Screening Among Injecting Drug Users Outside Treatment Settings: Implications for Research and Health Services," *Mental Health and Substance Use: Dual Diagnosis*, Vol. 1, No. 2, 2008, pp. 99–103.

American Hospital Association, *The State of the Behavioral Health Workforce: A Literature Review*, Chicago, 2016. As of October 2, 2018:
http://www.hpoe.org/Reports-HPOE/2016/aha_Behavioral_FINAL.pdf

Anderson, C. M., C. S. Robins, C. G. Greeno, H. Cahalane, V. C. Copeland, and R. M. Andrews, "Why Lower Income Mothers Do Not Engage with the Formal Mental Health Care System: Perceived Barriers to Care," *Qualitative Health Research*, Vol. 16, No. 7, 2006, pp. 926–943.

Anderson, J. K., E. Howarth, M. Vainre, P. B. Jones, and A. Humphrey, "A Scoping Literature Review of Service-Level Barriers for Access and Engagement With Mental Health Services for Children and Young People," *Children and Youth Services Review*, Vol. 77, 2017, pp. 164–176.

Ayangbayi, T., A. Okunade, M. Karakus, and T. Nianogo, "Characteristics of Hospital Emergency Room Visits for Mental and Substance Use Disorders," *Psychiatric Services*, Vol. 68, No. 4, 2017, pp. 408–410.

Babor, T. F., J. R. La Fuente, J. Saunders, and M. Grant, *AUDIT, the Alcohol Use Disorders Identification Test: Guidelines for Use in Primary Health Care*, Geneva: Substance Abuse Department, World Health Organization, 1992.

Barrowclough, C., G. Haddock, N. Tarrier, S. W. Lewis, J. Moring, R. O'Brien, N. Schofield, J. McGovern, "Randomized Controlled Trial of Motivational Interviewing, Cognitive Behavior Therapy, and Family Intervention for Patients with Comorbid Schizophrenia and Substance Use Disorders," *American Journal of Psychiatry*, Vol. 158, No. 10, 2001, pp. 1706–1713.

Belkin, G. S., J. Unutzer, R. C. Kessler, H. Verdeli, G. J. Raviola, K. Sachs, C. Oswald, and E. Eustache, "Scaling Up for the 'Bottom Billion': '5 x 5' Implementation of Community Mental Health Care in Low-Income Regions," *Psychiatric Services*, Vol. 62, No. 12, 2011, pp. 1494–1502.

Berner, M. M., L. Kriston, M. Bentele, and M. Härter, "The Alcohol Use Disorders Identification Test for Detecting At-Risk Drinking: A Systematic Review and Meta-Analysis," *Journal of Studies on Alcohol and Drugs*, Vol. 68, 2007, pp. 461–473.

Bisson, J. I., A. Ehlers, R. Matthews, S. Pilling, D. Richards, and S. Turner, "Psychological Treatments for Chronic Post-Traumatic Stress Disorder. Systematic Review and Meta-Analysis," *British Journal of Psychiatry*, Vol. 190, 2007, pp. 97–104.

Blevins, C. A., F. W. Weathers, M. T. Davis, T. K., Witte, and J. Domino, "The Posttraumatic Stress Disorder Checklist for DSM-5 (PCL-5): Development and Initial Psychometric Evaluation," *Journal of Traumatic Stress*, Vol. 28, No. 6, 2015, pp. 489–498.

Bolton, P., J. Bass, R. Neugebauer, H. Verdeli, K. F. Clougherty, P. Wickramaratne, L. Speelman, L. Ndogoni, and M. Weissman, "Group Interpersonal Psychotherapy for Depression in Rural Uganda—A Randomized Controlled Trial," *JAMA*, Vol. 289, No. 23, 2003, pp. 3117–3124.

Brody, D. J., L. A. Pratt, and J. P. Hughes, "Prevalence of Depression Among Adults Aged 20 and Over: United States, 2013–2016," Washington, D.C.: National Center for Health Statistics, February 2018. As of October 26, 2018: https://www.cdc.gov/nchs/data/databriefs/db303.pdf

Brummelte, S., and L. A. Galea, "Depression During Pregnancy and Postpartum: Contribution of Stress and Ovarian Hormones," *Progress in Neuro-Psychopharmacology and Biological Psychiatry*, Vol. 34, No. 5, 2010, pp. 766–776.

Burke, B. L., H. Arkowitz, and M. Menchola, "The Efficacy of Motivational Interviewing: A Meta-Analysis of Controlled Clinical Trials," *Journal of Consulting and Clinical Psychology*, Vol. 71, No. 5, 2003, pp. 843–861.

Cadigan, J. M., C. M. Lee, and M. E. Larimer, "Young Adult Mental Health: A Prospective Examination of Service Utilization, Perceived Unmet Service Needs, Attitudes, and Barriers to Service Use," *Prevention Science*, February 7, 2018.

Carlson, E., P. Palmieri, S. Smith, R. Kimerling, J. Ruzek, and T. Burling, *The Trauma History Screen (THS)*, measurement instrument, 2005.

Chan, Y. F., M. L. Dennis, and R. R. Funk, "Prevalence and Comorbidity of Major Internalizing and Externalizing Problems Among Adolescents and Adults Presenting to Substance Abuse Treatment," *Journal of Substance Abuse Treatment*, Vol. 34, No. 1, 2008, pp. 14–24.

Chang, C. K., R. D. Hayes, G. Perera, M. T. Broadbent, A. C. Fernandes, W. E. Lee, M. Hotopf, and R. Stewart, "Life Expectancy at Birth for People with Serious Mental Illness from a Secondary Mental Health Care Case Register in London," *PLos One*, Vol. 6, No. 5, 2011.

Chatterjee, S., S. Naik, S. John, H. Dabholkar, M. Balaji, M. Koschorke, M. Varghese, R. Thara, H. A. Weiss, P. Williams, P. McCrone, V. Patel, and G. Thornicroft, "Effectiveness of a Community-Based Intervention for People with Schizophrenia and Their Caregivers in India (COPSI): A Randomised Controlled Trial," *Lancet*, Vol. 383, No. 9926, 2014, pp. 1385–1394.

Chibanda, D., P. Mesu, L. Kajawu, F. Cowan, R. Araya, and M. A. Abas, "Problem-Solving Therapy for Depression and Common Mental Disorders in Zimbabwe: Piloting a Task-Shifting Primary Mental Health Care Intervention in a Population with a High Prevalence of People Living with HIV," *BMC Public Health*, Vol. 11, 2011, p. 828.

Chung, B., L. Jones, E. L. Dixon, J. Miranda, K. Wells, and Community Partners in Care Steering, "Using a Community Partnered Participatory Research Approach to Implement a Randomized Controlled Trial: Planning Community Partners in Care," *Journal of Health Care for the Poor and Underserved*, Vol. 21, No. 3, 2010, pp. 780–795.

City of New York, Office of the Mayor, "Report: Understanding New York City's Mental Health Challenge," press release, 2015. As of October 12, 2018: https://www1.nyc.gov/assets/home/downloads/pdf/press-releases/2015/thriveNYC_white_paper.pdf

Clement, S., E. Brohan, D. Jeffery, C. Henderson, S. L. Hatch, and G. Thornicroft, "Development and Psychometric Properties the Barriers to Access to Care Evaluation Scale (BACE) Related to People with Mental Ill Health," *BMC Psychiatry*, Vol. 12, No. 36, 2012.

Cuijpers, P., A. van Straten, and L. Warmerdam, "Behavioral Activation Treatments of Depression: A Meta-Analysis," *Clinical Psychology Review*, Vol. 27, No. 3, 2007, pp. 318–326.

Cunningham, M., and L. H. Zayas, "Reducing Depression in Pregnancy: Designing Multimodal Interventions," *Social Work*, Vol. 47, No. 2, 2002, pp. 114–123.

Cunningham, R. M., S. T. Chermack, M. A. Zimmerman, J. T. Shope, C. R. Bingham, F. C. Blow, and M. A. Walton, "Brief Motivational Interviewing Intervention for Peer Violence and Alcohol Use in Teens: One-Year Follow-Up," *Pediatrics*, Vol. 129, No. 6, 2012, pp. 1083–1090.

Cygan-Rehm, K., D. Kuehnle, and M. Oberfichtner, "Bounding the Causal Effect of Unemployment on Mental Health: Nonparametric Evidence from Four Countries," *Health Economics*, Vol. 26, No. 12, 2017, pp. 1844–1861.

de Roten, Y., G. Zimmermann, D. Ortega, and J. N. Despland, "Meta-Analysis of the Effects of MI Training on Clinicians' Behavior," *Journal of Substance Abuse Treatment*, Vol. 45, No. 2, 2013, pp. 155–162.

dos Santos, P. F., M. L. Wainberg, J. M. Caldas-de-Almeida, B. Saraceno, and J. D. Mari, "Overview of the Mental Health System in Mozambique: Addressing the Treatment Gap with a Task-Shifting Strategy in Primary Care," *International Journal of Mental Health Systems*, Vol. 10, 2016.

Edlund, M. J., B. M. Booth, and X. T. Han, "Who Seeks Care Where? Utilization of Mental Health and Substance Use Disorder Treatment in Two National Samples of Individuals with Alcohol Use Disorders," *Journal of Studies on Alcohol and Drugs*, Vol. 73, No. 4, 2012, pp. 635–646.

Elhai, J. D., W. Schweinle, and S. M. Anderson, "Reliability and Validity of the Attitudes Toward Seeking Professional Psychological Help Scale—Short Form," *Psychiatry Research*, Vol. 159, 2008, pp. 320–329.

Erickson, D., and N. Andrews, "Partnerships Among Community Development, Public Health, and Health Care Could Improve the Well-Being of Low-Income People," *Health Affairs*, Vol. 30, No. 11, 2011, pp. 2056–2063.

Evans-Lacko, S., K. Little, H. Meltzer, D. Rose, D. Rhydderch, C. Henderson, and G. Thornicroft, "Development and Psychometric Properties of the Mental Health Knowledge Schedule," *Canadian Journal of Psychiatry*, Vol. 55, No. 7, 2010, pp. 440–448.

Gopalan, G., L. Goldstein, K. Klingenstein, C. Sicher, C. Blake, and M. M. McKay, "Engaging Families into Child Mental Health Treatment: Updates and Special Considerations," *Journal of the Canadian Academy of Child and Adolescent Psychiatry*, Vol. 19, No. 3, 2010, pp. 182–196.

Gournellis, R., K. Tournikioti, G. Touloumi, C. Thomadakis, P. G. Michalopoulou, C. Christodoulou, A. Papadopoulou, and A. Douzenis, "Psychotic (Delusional) Depression and Suicidal Attempts: A Systematic Review and Meta-Analysis," *Acta Psychiatrica Scandanavica*, Vol. 137, No. 1, 2018, pp. 18–29.

Govindarajan, V., and R. Ramamurti, "Task Shifting Could Help Lower Costs in U.S. Health Care," *Harvard Business Review*, July 19, 2018.

Hadfield, H., and A. Wittkowski, "Women's Experiences of Seeking and Receiving Psychological and Psychosocial Interventions for Postpartum Depression: A Systematic Review and Thematic Synthesis of the Qualitative Literature," *Journal of Midwifery and Womens Health*, Vol. 62, No. 6, 2017, pp. 723–736.

Hahm, H. C., B. Cook, A. Ault-Brutus, and M. Alegria, "Intersection of Race-Ethnicity and Gender in Depression Care: Screening, Access, and Minimally Adequate Treatment," *Psychiatric Services*, Vol. 66, No. 3, 2015, pp. 258–264.

Hatzenbuehler, M. L., K. M. Keyes, W. E. Narrow, B. E. Grant, and D. S. Hasin, "Racial/Ethnic Disparities in Service Utilization for Individuals with Co-Occurring Mental Health and Substance Use Disorders in the General Population: Results from the National Epidemiologic Survey on Alcohol and Related Conditions," *Journal of Clinical Psychiatry*, Vol. 69, No. 7, 2008, pp. 1112–1121.

Hingson, R., and J. Howland, "Alcohol as a Risk Factor for Injury or Death Resulting from Accidental Falls: A Review of the Literature," *Journal of Studies on Alcohol*, Vol. 48, No. 3, 1987, pp. 212–219.

Hofmann, S. G., and J. A. Smits, "Cognitive-Behavioral Therapy for Adult Anxiety Disorders: A Meta-Analysis of Randomized Placebo-Controlled Trials," *Journal of Clinical Psychiatry*, Vol. 69, No. 4, 2008, pp. 621–632.

Hohmna, M., N. Doran, and I. Koutsenok, "Motivational Interviewing Training for Juvenile Correctional Staff in California: One Year Initial Outcomes," *Journal of Offender Rehabilitation*, Vol. 48, No. 7, 2009, pp. 635–648.

Huang, K. Y., J. Nakigudde, E. Calzada, M. J. Boivin, G. Ogedegbe, and Brotman, L. M., "Implementing an Early Childhood School-Based Mental Health Promotion Intervention in Low-Resource Ugandan Schools: Study Protocol for a Cluster Randomized Controlled Trial," *Trials*, Vol. 15, No. 471, 2014.

Jensen, C. D., C. C. Cushing, B. S. Aylward, J. T. Craig, D. M. Sorell, and R. G. Steele, "Effectiveness of Motivational Interviewing Interventions for Adolescent Substance Use Behavior Change: A Meta-Analytic Review," *Journal of Consulting and Clinical Psychology*, Vol. 79, No. 4, 2011, pp. 433–440.

Kagee, A., A. C. Tsai, C. Lund, and M. Tomlinson, "Screening for Common Mental Disorders in Low Resource Settings: Reasons for Caution and a Way Forward," *International Health*, Vol. 5, No. 1, 2013, pp. 11–14.

Kakuma, R., H. Minas, N. van Ginneken, M. R. Dal Poz, K. Desiraju, J. E. Morris, S. Saxena, and R. M. Scheffler, "Human Resources for Mental Health Care: Current Situation and Strategies for Action," *Lancet*, Vol. 378, No. 9803, 2011, pp. 1654–1663.

Kataoka, S. H., L. Zhang, and K. B. Wells, "Unmet Need for Mental Health Care Among U.S. Children: Variation by Ethnicity and Insurance Status," *American Journal of Psychiatry*, Vol. 159, No. 9, 2002, pp. 1548–1555.

Kazdin, A. E., and S. M. Rabbitt, "Novel Models for Delivering Mental Health Services and Reducing the Burdens of Mental Illness," *Clinical Psychological Science*, Vol. 1, No. 2, 2013, pp. 170–191.

Kessler R.C., P. R. Barker, L. J. Colpe, J. F. Epstein, J. C. Gfroerer, E. Hiripi, M. J. Howes, S. L. Normand, R. W. Manderscheid, E. E. Walters, and A. M. Zaslavsky, "Screening for Serious Mental Illness in the General Population," *Archives of General Psychiatry*, Vol. 60, 2003, pp. 184–189.

Kessler, R. C., S. Heeringa, M. D. Lakoma, M., Petukhova, A. E. Rupp, M. Schoenbaum, P. S. Wang, and A. M. Zaslavsky, "Individual and Societal Effects of Mental Disorders on Earnings in the United States: Results from the National Comorbidity Survey Replication," *American Journal of Psychiatry*, Vol. 165, No. 6, 2008, pp. 703–711.

Kroenke, K., T. W. Strine, R. L. Spitzer, J. B. Williams, J. T. Berry, and A. H. Mokdad, "The PHQ-8 as a Measure of Current Depression in the General Population," *Journal of Affective Disorders*, Vol. 114, No. 1, 2009, pp. 163–173.

Krysinska, K., and D. Lester, "Post-Traumatic Stress Disorder and Suicide Risk: A Systematic Review," *Archives of Suicide Research*, Vol. 14, No. 1, 2010, pp. 1–23.

Kvalevaag, A. L., P. G. Ramchandani, O. Hove, J. Assmus, M. Eberhard-Gran, and E. Biringer, "Paternal Mental Health and Socioemotional and Behavioral Development in Their Children," *Pediatrics*, Vol. 131, No. 2, 2013, pp. e463–e469.

Lazear, K. J., S. A. Pires, M. R. Isaacs, P. Chaulk, and L. Huang, "Depression Among Low-Income Women of Color: Qualitative Findings from Cross-Cultural Focus Groups," *Journal of Immigrant and Minority Health*, Vol. 10, No. 2, 2008, pp. 127–133.

Legha, R., E. Eustache, T. Therosme, K. Boyd, F. Reginald, G. Hilaire, S. Daimyo, G. Jerome, H. Verdeli, and G. Raviola, "Taskshifting: Translating Theory into Practice to Build a Community Based Mental Health Care System in Rural Haiti," *Intervention*, Vol. 13, No. 3, 2015, pp. 248–267.

Lehman, W. E. K., J. M. Greener, and D. D. Simpson, "Assessing Organizational Readiness for Change," *Journal of Substance Abuse Treatment*, Vol. 22, 2002, pp. 197–209.

Liem, J. H., K. Lustig, and C. Dillon, "Depressive Symptoms and Life Satisfaction Among Emerging Adults: A Comparison of High School Dropouts and Graduates," *Journal of Adult Development*, Vol. 17, No. 1, 2010, pp. 33–43.

Link, B. G., F. T. Cullen, A. Struening, P. E. Shrout, and B. P. Dohrenwend, "A Modified Labelling Theory Approach to Mental Disorders: An Empirical Assessment," *American Sociological Review*, Vol. 54, No. 3, 1989, pp. 400–423.

Löwe, B., O. Decker, S. Müller, E. Brähler, D. Schellberg, W. Herzog, and P. Y. Herzberg, "Validation and Standardization of the Generalized Anxiety Disorder Screener (GAD-7) in the General Population," *Medical Care*, Vol. 46, No. 3, 2008, pp. 266–274.

Lubman, D. I., L. Hides, A. Scaffidi, K. Elkins, M. Stevens, and R. Marks, "Implementing Mental Health Screening Within a Youth Alcohol and Other Drug Service," *Mental Health and Substance Use: Dual Diagnosis*, Vol. 1, No. 3, 2008, pp. 254–261.

Lukens, E., and W. R. McFarlane, "Psychoeducation as Evidence-Based Practice: Considerations for Practice, Research, and Policy," *Brief Treatment and Crisis Intervention*, Vol. 4, No. 3, 2004, pp. 205–225.

Lundahl, B., and B. L. Burke, "The Effectiveness and Applicability of Motivational Interviewing: A Practice-Friendly Review of Four Meta-Analyses," *Journal of Clinical Psychology*, Vol. 65, No. 11, 2009, pp. 1232–1245.

Matsuzaka, C. T., M. Wainberg, A. N. Pala, E. V. Hoffmann, B. M. Coimbra, R. F. Braga, A. C. Sweetland, and M. F. Mello, "Task Shifting Interpersonal Counseling for Depression: A Pragmatic Randomized Controlled Trial in Primary Care," *BMC Psychiatry*, Vol. 17, 2017.

Maynard, B. R., C. P. Salas-Wright, and M. G. Vaughn, "High School Dropouts in Emerging Adulthood: Substance Use, Mental Health Problems, and Crime," *Community Mental Health Journal*, Vol. 51, No. 3, 2015, pp. 289–299.

McHugh, R. K., and D. H. Barlow, "The Dissemination and Implementation of Evidence-Based Psychological Treatments. A Review of Current Efforts," *American Psychologist*, Vol. 65, No. 2, 2010, pp. 73–84.

Mehta, P., A. Brown, B. Chung, F. Jones, L. Tang, J. Gilmore, J. Miranda, and K. Wells, "Community Partners in Care: 6-Month Outcomes of Two Quality Improvement Depression Care Interventions in Male Participants," *Ethnicity and Disease*, Vol. 27, No. 3, 2017, pp. 223–232.

Mental Health First Aid USA, *Mental Health First Aid USA—Certification Standards*, 2012. As of October 2, 2018:
https://www.nationalcouncildocs.net/wp-content/uploads/2013/10/MHFA-USA-Certification-Standards-Updated-Aug-2012.pdf

Mental Health First Aid USA, "Certification Process," webpage, 2018. As of October 2, 2018:
https://www.mentalhealthfirstaid.org/become-an-instructor/certification-process/

Mericle, A. A., V. M. Ta Park, P. Holck, and A. M. Arria, "Prevalence, Patterns, and Correlates of Co-Occurring Substance Use and Mental Disorders in the United States: Variations by Race/Ethnicity," *Comprehensive Psychiatry*, Vol. 53, No. 6, 2012, pp. 657–665.

Metrik, J., K. Jackson, S. S. Bassett, M. J. Zvolensky, K., Seal, and B. Borsari, "The Mediating Roles of Coping, Sleep, and Anxiety Motives in Cannabis Use and Problems Among Returning Veterans with PTSD and MDD," *Psychology of Addictive Behaviors*, Vol. 30, No. 7, 2016, pp. 743–754.

Miller, W. R., and S. Rollnick, *Motivational Interviewing in Health Care*, New York: Guilford Press, 2008.

Miller, W. R., and S. Rollnick, *Motivational Interviewing, Helping People Change*, 3rd ed., New York: Guilford Press, 2013.

Miranda, J., J. Y. Chung, B. L. Green, J. Krupnick, J. Siddique, D. A. Revicki, and T. Belin, "Treating Depression in Predominantly Low-Income Young Minority Women: A Randomized Controlled Trial," *JAMA*, Vol. 290, No. 1, 2003, pp. 57–65.

Motivational Interviewing Network of Trainers, homepage, undated. As of October 2, 2018: http://www.motivationalinterviewing.org

Moyers, T. B., T. Martin, J. K. Manuel, S. M. L. Hendrickson, and W. R. Miller, "Assessing Competence in the Use of Motivational Interviewing," *Journal of Substance Abuse Treatment*, Vol. 28, No. 1, 2005, pp. 19–26.

Muntaner, C., W. W. Eaton, C. Diala, R. C. Kessler, and P. D. Sorlie, "Social Class, Assets, Organizational Control and the Prevalence of Common Groups of Psychiatric Disorders," *Social Science & Medicine*, Vol. 47, No. 12, 1998, pp. 2043–2053.

New York City Department of Health and Mental Hygiene, "Mental Health First Aid Trainings," webpage, undated. As of October 4, 2018: https://www1.nyc.gov/site/doh/health/health-topics/mental-health-first-aid.page

Olsson, M. O., L. Bradvik, A. Ojehagen, and A. Hakansson, "Risk Factors for Unnatural Death: Fatal Accidental Intoxication, Undetermined Intent and Suicide: Register Follow-Up in a Criminal Justice Population with Substance Use Problems," *Drug Alcohol and Dependence*, Vol. 162, 2016, pp. 176–181.

Patel, V., G. S. Belkin, A. Chockalingam, J. Cooper, S. Saxena, and J. Unutzer, "Grand Challenges: Integrating Mental Health Services into Priority Health Care Platforms," *PLoS Medicine*, Vol 10, No. 5, 2013.

Pekkala, E., and L. Merinder, "Psychoeducation for Schizophrenia," *Cochrane Database of Systemic of Review*, Vol. 2, 2002.

Penninx, B. W., S. Leveille, L. Ferrucci, J. T. van Eijk, and J. M. Guralnik, "Exploring the Effect of Depression on Physical Disability: Longitudinal Evidence from the Established Populations for Epidemiologic Studies of the Elderly," *American Journal of Public Health,* Vol. 89, No. 9, 1999, pp. 1346–1352.

Petrenko, C. L., S. E. Culhane, E. F. Garrido, and H. N. Taussig, "Do Youth in Out-Of-Home Care Receive Recommended Mental Health and Educational Services Following Screening Evaluations?" *Children and Youth Services Review,* Vol. 33, No. 10, 2011, pp. 1911–1918.

Ramchand, R., L. Ayer, L. Geyer, A. Kofner, and L. Burgette, "Non-Commissioned Officers' Perspectives on Identifying, Caring for, and Referring Soldiers at Risk for Suicide," *Psychiatric Services,* Vol. 66, 2015, pp. 1057–1063.

RAND Corporation, *Connections to Care (C2C): Evaluating an Initiative Integrating Mental Health Supports into Social Service Settings,* Santa Monica, Calif., CP-857, 2017. As of October 2, 2018:
https://www.rand.org/pubs/corporate_pubs/CP857-2017-01.html

Roll, J. M., J. Kennedy, M. Tran, and D. Howell, "Disparities in Unmet Need for Mental Health Services in the United States, 1997–2010," *Psychiatric Services,* Vol. 64, No. 1, 2013, pp. 80–82.

Roy-Byrne, P., M. G. Craske, G. Sullivan, R. D. Rose, M. J. Edlund, A. J. Lang, A. Bystritsky, S. S. Welch, D. A. Chavira, D. Golinelli, L. Campbell-Sills, C. D. Sherbourne, and M. B. Stein, "Delivery of Evidence-Based Treatment for Multiple Anxiety Disorders in Primary Care: A Randomized Controlled Trial," *JAMA,* Vol. 303, No. 19, 2010, pp. 1921–1928.

Santiago, C. D., S. Kaltman, and J. Miranda, "Poverty and Mental Health: How Do Low-Income Adults and Children Fare in Psychotherapy?" *Journal of Clinical Psychology,* Vol. 69, No. 2, 2013, pp. 115–126.

Sarason, I. G., J. H. Johnson, and J. M. Siegel, "Assessing the Impact of Life Changes: Development of the Life Experiences Survey," *Journal of Consulting and Clinical Psychology,* Vol. 46, 1978, pp. 932–946.

Scheirer, M. A., and J. W. Dearing, "An Agenda for Research on the Sustainability of Public Health Programs," *American Journal of Public Health,* Vol. 101, No. 11, 2011, pp. 2059–2067.

Schwalbe, C. S., H. Y. Oh, and A. Zweben, "Sustaining Motivational Interviewing: A Meta-Analysis of Training Studies," *Addiction,* Vol. 109, No. 8, 2014, pp. 1287–1294.

Shaffer, D., A. N. N. Garland, V. Vieland, M. Underwood, and C. Busner, "The Impact of Curriculum-Based Suicide Prevention Programs for Teenagers," *Journal of the American Academy of Child and Adolescent Psychiatry,* Vol. 30, No. 4, 1991, pp. 588–596.

Shear, K., E. Frank, P. R. Houck, and C. F. Reynolds, 3rd, "Treatment of Complicated Grief: A Randomized Controlled Trial," *JAMA*, Vol. 293, No. 21, 2005, pp. 2601–2608.

Shippee, N. D., B. H. Rosen, K. B. Angstman, M. E. Fuentes, R. S. DeJesus, S. M. Bruce, and M. D. Williams, "Baseline Screening Tools as Indicators for Symptom Outcomes and Health Services Utilization in a Collaborative Care Model for Depression in Primary Care: A Practice-Based Observational Study," *General Hospital Psychiatry*, Vol. 36, No. 6, 2014, pp. 563–569.

Skevington, S., M. Lotfy, and K. O'Connell, "The World Health Organization's WHOQOL-BREF Quality of Life Assessment: Psychometric Properties and Results of the International Field Trial: A Report from the WHOQOL Group," *Quality of Life Research*, Vol. 13, 2004, p. 299.

Smith, J. L., K. M. Carpenter, P. C. Amrhein, A. C. Brooks, D. Levin, E. A. Schreiber, L. A. Travaglini, M. C. Hu, and E. V. Nunes, "Training Substance Abuse Clinicians in Motivational Interviewing Using Live Supervision Via Teleconferencing," *Journal of Consulting of Clinical Psychology*, Vol. 80, No. 3, 2012, pp. 450–464.

Spitzer, R. L., K. Kroenke, J. B. Williams, and B. Löwe, "A Brief Measure For Assessing Generalized Anxiety Disorder: The GAD-7," *Archives of Internal Medicine*, Vol. 166, No. 10, 2006, pp. 1092–1097.

Substance Abuse and Mental Health Services Administration, *Results from the 2002 National Survey on Drug Use and Health: National Findings*, Rockville, Md., National Household Survey on Drug Abuse Series H-22, Publication No. SMA 03-3836, 2003.

Thomas, A. C., and P. K. Staiger, "Introducing Mental Health and Substance Use Screening into a Community-Based Health Service in Australia: Usefulness and Implications for Service Change," *Health and Social Care in the Community*, Vol. 20, No. 6, 2012, pp. 635–644.

Thomas, K. C., A. R. Ellis, T. R. Konrad, C. E. Holzer, and J. P. Morrissey, "County-Level Estimates of Mental Health Professional Shortage in the United States," *Psychiatric Services*, Vol. 60, No. 10, 2009, pp. 1323–1328.

Tompkins, T. L., and J. Witt, "The Short-Term Effectiveness of a Suicide Prevention Gatekeeper Training Program in a College Setting with Residence Life Advisers," *Journal of Primary Prevention*, Vol. 30, 2009, pp. 131–149.

Towe, V. L., L. Leviton, A. Chandra, J. C. Sloan, M. Tait, and T. Orleans, "Cross-Sector Collaborations and Partnerships: Essential Ingredients to Help Shape Health and Well-Being," *Health Affairs*, Vol. 35, No. 11, 2016, pp. 1964–1969.

Ustun, T. B., N. Kostanjsek, S. Chatterji, and J. Rehm, eds., *Measuring Health and Disability: Manual for WHO Disability Assessment Schedule,* Geneva, Switzerland: World Health Organization, 2010.

van Ginneken, N., P. Tharyan, S. Lewin, G. N. Rao, S. M. Meera, J. Pian, S. Chandrashekar, and V. Patel, "Non-Specialist Health Worker Interventions for the Care of Mental, Neurological and Substance-Abuse Disorders in Low- and Middle-Income Countries," *Cochrane Database of Systemic of Review,* Vol. 11, 2013.

Vigo, D., G. Thornicroft, and R. Atun, "Estimating the True Global Burden of Mental Illness," *Lancet Psychiatry,* Vol. 3, No. 7, 2016, pp. 171–178.

Wang, P. S., M. Lane, M. Olfson, H. A. Pincus, K. B., Wells, and R. C. Kessler, "Twelve-Month Use of Mental Health Services in the United States: Results from the National Comorbidity Survey Replication," *Archives of General Psychiatry,* Vol. 62, No. 6, 2005, pp. 629–640.

Watkins, K. E., S. B. Hunter, S. L. Wenzel, W. Tu, S. M. Paddock, A. Griffin, and P. Ebener, "Prevalence and Characteristics of Clients with Co-Occurring Disorders in Outpatient Substance Abuse Treatment," *American Journal of Drug and Alcohol Abuse,* Vol. 30, No. 4, 2004, pp. 749–764.

Wong, Eunice C., Rebecca L. Collins, and Jennifer L. Cerully, *Reviewing the Evidence Base for Mental Health First Aid: Is There Support for Its Use with Key Target Populations in California?* Santa Monica, Calif.: RAND Corporation, RR-972-CMHSA, 2015. As of October 2, 2018:
https://www.rand.org/pubs/research_reports/RR972.html

World Health Organization, *Prevention of Mental Disorders: Effective Interventions and Policy Options,* Geneva, 2004. As of October 4, 2018:
http://www.who.int/mental_health/evidence/en/prevention_of_mental_disorders_sr.pdf

Wyman, P. A., C. Hendricks Brown, J. Inman, W. Cross, K. Schmeelk-Cone, J. Guo, and J. B. Pena, "Randomized Trial of a Gatekeeper Program for Suicide Prevention: 1-Year Impact on Secondary School Staff," *Journal of Consulting and Clinical Psychology,* Vol. 76, 2008, pp. 104–115.

Yudko, E., O. Lozhkina, and A. Fouts, "A Comprehensive Review of the Psychometric Properties of the Drug Abuse Screening Test," *Journal of Substance Abuse Treatment,* Vol. 32, No. 2, 2007, pp. 189–198.

Zalewski, M., S. H. Goodman, P. M. Cole, and K. A. McLaughlin, "Clinical Considerations When Treating Adults Who Are Parents," *Clinical Psychology—Science and Practice,* Vol. 24, No. 4, 2017, pp. 370–388.